Comprehensive Guide
to Neurosurgical Conditions

W0051313

Abhishek Agrawal • Gavin Britz
Editors

Comprehensive Guide to Neurosurgical Conditions

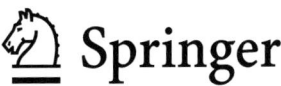 Springer

Editors

Abhishek Agrawal, M.D
Department of Neurosurgery
and Radiology
Brigham and Women's Hospital
Harvard Medical School
Boston, MA
USA

Gavin Britz
Department of Neurosurgery
Methodist Neurological Institute
Houston, TX
USA

ISBN 978-3-319-06565-6   ISBN 978-3-319-06566-3   (eBook)
DOI 10.1007/978-3-319-06566-3
Springer Cham Heidelberg New York Dordrecht London

Library of Congress Control Number: 2014958080

Printed on acid-free paper

Springer is part of Springer Science+Business Media (www.springer.com)

Preface

Patients with neurosurgical conditions are almost always referred from either primary care physicians, neurologists, internist, or a specialist in family medicine. This two-volume guide will answer commonly asked questions about neurosurgical conditions related to brain and spinal cord, in an attempt to fill in the gap and answer numerous questions that arise after a diagnosis is made, explaining the basics of neurosurgical disease spectrum and their management options.

Comprehensive Guide to Neurosurgical Conditions (*Volume I*) updates the reader on basic neuroanatomy and physiology, including general neurosurgical conditions, ideal neurosurgical and intensive care unit set up, second opinion, brain death, and organ donation in a comprehensive and concise manner.

Comprehensive Guide which is part of a book set including *Emergency Approaches to Neurosurgical Conditions* (*Volume II*) delves into different kinds of complex brain surgeries and focuses on the surgical aspect of neurosurgical conditions, including management of tumors, aneurysms, and pediatric conditions in chapters written by reputed neurosurgeons in their allied subspecialty.

This two-volume book set also aims to replace "excess-information" obtained on the internet about a particular neurosurgical disease, which may be too overwhelming, not complied properly, not updated, or may be misinterpreted, misunderstood, or irrelevant for that particular disease. This concise book is intended not only for neurologists or neurosurgeons who have direct patient interaction but also for brain surgery patients and their families, medical students, paramedics, nurse practitioners, physician assistants, health planners, residents, and fellows who are already trained or in training, to get a quick glimpse of neurosurgical conditions encountered on a day-to-day basis.

Boston, MA, USA   Abhishek Agrawal
Houston, TX, USA   Gavin Britz

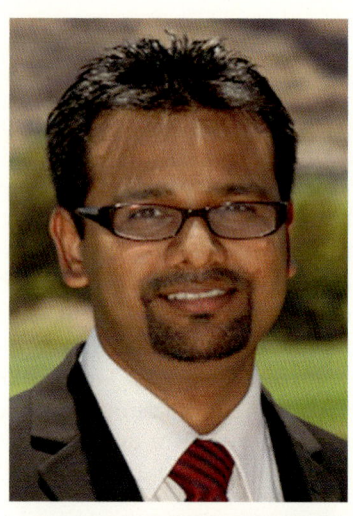

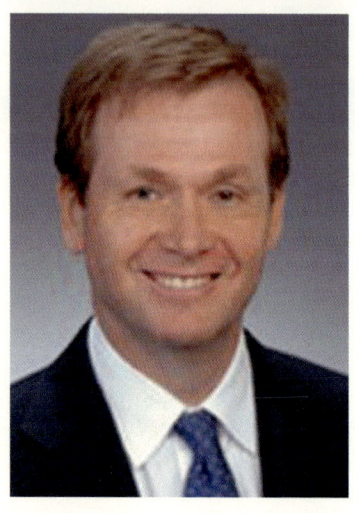

Acknowledgments

The key to success of any project depends upon the inputs and guidance received from persons associated with the project. Fortunately for us, there was encouragement, guidance, and support from all quarters of life.

Great are those who teach and inspire. They deserve gratitude which can be expressed at a time like this. Our inestimable gratitude goes to our colleagues and authors who spend their precious time contributing chapters for this book.

We are also thankful to our assistant, Peggy Kelly, who managed to keep track of the chapters and authors. In addition, we would like to express our gratitude to Melissa Morton, Julia Megginson, and R. Nithyatharani from Springer Publishers for their collegiality.

Behind all this is the unconditional support, motivation, and encouragement from our family members, parents, and children who have always been a source of strength and inspiration.

Abhishek Agrawal
Gavin Britz

Contents

Contributors

Wenya Linda Bi, MD, PhD   Department of Neurosurgery, Brigham and Women's Hospital, Boston, MA, USA

Harjus S. Birk   School of Medicine, University of California, San Francisco, San Francisco, CA, USA

Tene Cage   Department of Neurosurgery, University of California, San Francisco, San Francisco, CA, USA

E. Antonio Chiocca, MD, PhD   Department of Neurosurgery, Brigham and Women's Hospital, Boston, MA, USA

Purvi Desai, MD   Department of Physical Medicine and Rehabilitation, Houston Methodist Hospital, Houston, TX, USA

David S. Enterline, MD, FACR   Department of Radiology, Duke University, Durham, NC, USA

Kai Frerichs, MD   Department of Neurosurgery, Brigham and Women's Hospital, Boston, MA, USA

Leo Galvin, MD, MRCPI, FFRRCSI   Department of Radiology, Duke University, Durham, NC, USA

Sankalp Gokhale   Departments of Neurology, Duke University Medical Center, Durham, NC, USA

Robert G. Grossman, MD   Department of Neurosurgery, Houston Methodist Hospital, Houston, TX, USA

Caitlin Hoffman, MD   Department of Neurological Surgery, Weill Cornell Medical College, New York, NY, USA

Ibrahim Hussain, MD Department of Neurological Surgery, Weill Cornell Medical College, New York, NY, USA

Zakiyah Kadry Division of Transplantation, Department of Surgery, Penn State Hershey Medical Center, Hershey, PA, USA

Teresa Kaldis, MD Methodist Rehabilitation Associates, Houston Methodist Hospital, Houston, TX, USA

Rahul Kapoor, BS Department of Neurological Surgery, Weill Cornell Medical College, New York, NY, USA

Kathryn Kerrigan, MSN, FNP-BC Houston Methodist Neurological Institute, Houston, TX, USA

John P. Kirkpatrick, MD, PhD Department of Radiation Oncology, Duke University Medical Center, Durham, NC, USA

Department of Surgery, Duke University Medical Center, Durham, NC, USA

Duke Cancer Institute, Duke University Medical Center, Durham, NC, USA

Michel Kliot, MD Department of Neurosurgery, University of Northwestern Feinberg School of Medicine, Chicago, IL, USA

Kristin Lewis, NP Department of Neurosurgery, Brigham and Women's Hospital, Boston, MA, USA

John C. Lohlun Division of Transplantation, Department of Surgery, Penn State Hershey Medical Center, Hershey, PA, USA

David L. McDonagh Departments of Neurology, Duke University Medical Center, Durham, NC, USA

Departments of Anesthesiology, Duke University Medical Center, Durham, NC, USA

Jessica McElheny Departments of Neurology, Duke University Medical Center, Durham, NC, USA

Neal Mehan, MD Department of Neurosurgery, Hofstra North Shore LIJ School of Medicine, Manhasset, NY, USA

Raj K. Narayan, MD Department of Neurosurgery, Hofstra North Shore LIJ School of Medicine, Manhasset, NY, USA

Shahid M. Nimjee, MD, PhD Division of Neurosurgery, Department of Radiology, Duke University Medical Center, Durham, NC, USA

Rob Parrish, MD, PhD Department of Neurosurgery, Houston Methodist Hospital, Houston, TX, USA

Kenneth Podell, PhD Houston Methodist Concussion Center, Houston, TX, USA

David B. Rosenfield, MD EMG and Motor Control Laboratory, Speech and Language Center, Neurological Institute, Houston Methodist Hospital, Weill Medical College of Cornell University, Houston, TX, USA

Philip Stieg, PhD, MD Department of Neurological Surgery, Weill Cornell Medical College, New York, NY, USA

John J. Volpi, MD Department of Neurology, Houston Methodist Neurological Institute, Houston, TX, USA

Katherine E. Wood, BS Houston Methodist, Houston, TX, USA

Fang-Fang Yin, PhD Department of Radiation Oncology, Duke University Medical Center, Durham, NC, USA

Duke Cancer Institute, Duke University Medical Center, Durham, NC, USA

Chapter 1
Basic Neuro Anatomy

Rob Parrish

Anatomy, one would think, does not change. After all anatomically we are much the same as we were tens of thousands of years ago. What continues to change is our understanding of the form and function of our anatomy. The advent of current imaging techniques helps us understand the relationship between physical and structural anatomy and function. The nervous system has been particularly difficult for anatomists, physiologists, and physicians to investigate. The brain and spinal cord are enclosed in boney compartments, the brain in the skull and the spinal cord in the spinal canal surrounded by the bones of the spine. The nerves that project from and to the nervous system are found throughout the body. Their relationships and how they control muscles and organ systems is a continued area of research. Needless to say volumes have been and continue to be written about Neuro Anatomy. Many scholarly books are available from the usual sources. We attempt here to form the most very basic understanding of the form and function of the brain, spinal cord and peripheral nerves as a basis for understanding subsequent chapters on disease processes that affect the nervous system's form and function.

R. Parrish, MD, PhD
Department of Neurosurgery, Houston Methodist Hospital,
6560 Fannin Street, Suite 944, Houston, TX 77030, USA
e-mail: rparrish@houstonmethodist.org

A. Agrawal, G. Britz (eds.), *Comprehensive Guide to Neurosurgical Conditions*, DOI 10.1007/978-3-319-06566-3_1,
© Springer International Publishing Switzerland 2015

The human brain weighs about 3 lb which is less than 2 % of an average adult body weight. Yet the brain receives more than 15 % of the blood supply implying significant energy requirements even at rest. We divide the brain into an upper part, called the cerebrum, a lower part, called the cerebellum and part that is connected to almost everything, called the brain stem. The Cerebrum is further divided into right and left halves, the hemispheres and further divided into lobes, frontal, parietal, occipital and temporal. The cerebrum, the top part of the brain is the part of the brain that is responsible for thought processes, emotions, movement control, sensory perception, memory and vision. The right half of the cerebrum controls the left half of the body and the left half controls the right half of the body. For right handed people we speak of the left hemisphere being dominant. The dominant hemisphere is where most language functions reside. The "non-dominant" side is credited with math, music and creativity among other functions. The entire neural cavity, the cranium or head and the spinal column comprise the neural axis and is surrounded by a thin filmy membrane called the Arachnoid and a thicker membrane called the Dura Mater, commonly referred to as the Dura. We speak of spaces within the neural axis (brain, spinal cord, and spinal nerves) regarding these membranes. Thus something that is outside the arachnoid but under the dura is said to be sub-dural where as something that is inside the Arachnoid but outside the brain is said to be sub-arachnoid.

Within the Cerebrum are fluid filled cavities called the ventricles. The fluid in the cavities is the Cerebro Spinal Fluid or CSF. Each of the hemispheres of the cerebrum has a ventricle, the lateral ventricle. The CSF manufactured in the lateral ventricles flows into a central ventricle, called the Third Ventricle, then through a small aperture called the Aqueduct into the Fourth Ventricle that lies between the Cerebellum and Brain Stem.

The Frontal Lobe of the brain, appropriately, is the front part of the Cerebrum. It is involved in higher or executive functioning. It has association thought process input that helps us recognize the consequences of our actions. Thus someone with damage to both frontal lobes may have difficulty with impulse control and might speak his or her mind without recognizing the impact that thought might have on relationships. People who have had brain operations on both sides or closed head injuries with hemorrhages in both frontal lobes are susceptible to this behaviour problem. Yet, most of the executive function lies in the dominant frontal lobe, the left, for most right handed people. Thus, removal of a tumor or other lesion from the non-dominant anterior portion of the frontal lobe usually has little effect on behavior but may show changes on detailed neuropsychological testing. The posterior portion of the frontal lobe has to do with motor function and damage to this area leads to loss of motor function on the opposite side of the body. The posterior border of the frontal lobe is a deep groove in the brain called the central sulcus. It is approximately half way between the posterior tip and the anterior tip of the Cerebrum.

The Parietal Lobe lies behind the Frontal Lobe and the Central Sulcus. The Parietal Lobe is involved with sensation and interpreting and processing that information. Sensory input from the entire body comes to the Parietal lobe through a structure in the center of the brain called the Thalamus. The information is processed and there are connections throughout the brain to interpret the input. This includes input from the cranial nerves and thus the Parietal Lobe is involved in understanding language and appreciation of music among other important sensory functions.

The Cerebellum lies behind the Brain stem and beneath the occipital lobe of the cerebrum. The Cerebellum is separated from the Cerebrum by a thick membrane called the Tentorium which is made of Dura Mater. The Cerebellum controls motor coordination. It has some complex higher functions even involving speech but we think of it mostly as being involved with fine tuning movements. It is thus important in balance, walking and all those other motor functions. The right half of the cerebellum is mostly involved with the right half of the body and the left half the left side. The central part of the cerebellum is involved with posture and damage to the central portion of the cerebellum can make it difficult for a patient to even sit erect, much less stand. As mentioned above the Cerebellum is behind the Fourth Ventricle. Therefore, lesions such as tumors or hemorrhages in the Cerebellum can obstruct the flow of CSF and create a dangerous and life threatening situation.

The brain stem is a bundle of nerve cells and fibers that ties the nervous system together. The Brain Stem connects with the Cerebrum above and the spinal cord below. With few exceptions, (vision and sense of smell) all the input and output from the Cerebrum goes through the brain stem. Automatic functions such as breathing, sweating, tearing, and even food digestions are under Brain Stem control. We call these autonomic functions. The Brain Stem also has direct connections to the outside with nerves that go to and from the sensory and motor functions of the head. These nerves are called cranial nerves and historically are numbered one through twelve in more or less a front of the Cerebrum to the bottom of the Brain Stem numbering system. See Table 1.1 for a list of the cranial nerves and their functions. The Brain Stem extends from just beneath the Cerebrum where it is connected to the Thalamus to the base of the skull where it is connected to the Spinal Cord at the opening in the bottom of the skull, the Foramen Magnum.

The Spinal Cord connects the brain to the body. Muscle movements originate in the Cerebrum and the signal passes through the brain stem, modulated by the Cerebellum, into the spinal cord and out the nerves to muscles in the body. Correspondingly sensation of touch and pain come from the periphery, skin, bones and muscle and are transmitted via the spinal cord to the brain. The spinal cord begins at the Foramen Magnum and in the adult ends at the upper portion of the lumbar spine, the portion of the spine that makes up the low back. Problems that affect the spinal cord cause changes distal to the problem. That is, a problem in the neck can cause loss of sensation and motor function in the entire

TABLE 1.1 Cranial nerves and their function

(i)	Olfactory nerve	Sense of smell
(ii)	Optic nerves	Vision
(iii)	Oculomotor nerve	Eye movement and opens the eye
(iv)	Trochlear nerve	Eye movement
(v)	Trigeminal nerve	Sensation to the face and muscles of mastication
(vi)	Abducens nerve	Eye movement
(vii)	Facial nerve	Movement of facial muscles
(viii)	Vestibulocochlear nerve	Hearing and balance
(ix)	Glossopharyngeal nerve	Sensation in the back of the tongue and throat and some movement of throat muscles. Also sensation to some of the ear drum and canal
(x)	Vagus nerve	Overlaps function with the Glossopharyngeal nerve and also innervates the abdominal and thoracic cavities. It has strong connections in the brain stem related to blood pressure control and food digestion
(xi)	Accessory nerve	Innervates the sternocleidomastoid muscle and trapezius muscles which elevate the shoulders
(xii)	Hypoglossal nerve	Movement of the tongue

body. The nerves that come from the spinal cord innervate muscles of the body. Nerves that come from the Cervical portion of the spinal cord go to muscles in the arms and hands. Nerves that exit from the lower spinal cord go to muscles of the lower trunk and legs.

Chapter 2
Basic Neurology

John J. Volpi

Neurology is the study of the brain and the nervous system. Practically every disease effects the nervous system, and therefore almost all doctors, nurses, pharmacists, and other health professionals treat neurological conditions in one way or another. Common conditions, such as headaches, are caused by neurological problems as are life threatening conditions like strokes, seizures, and brain tumors. In this chapter, concepts about the basic organization and function of the nervous system will be covered. We will start, though, with a discussion of the common members of the treating team to better understand their roles in treating a patient with a neurological disease.

Understanding the Care Team

What Is a Neurologist?

A neurologist is a doctor who specializes in the medical treatment of neurological disorders. A neurologist does not perform surgery, but often helps to decide when surgery is

J.J. Volpi, MD
Department of Neurology, Houston Methodist Neurological Institute, 6560 Fannin Suite 802, Houston, TX 77030, USA
e-mail: jjvolpi@houstonmethodist.org

A. Agrawal, G. Britz (eds.), *Comprehensive Guide to Neurosurgical Conditions*, DOI 10.1007/978-3-319-06566-3_2, © Springer International Publishing Switzerland 2015

necessary and what type of surgeon to request. Neurologist are called to treat critically ill patients with conditions such as stroke, seizures, infections of the brain, sudden nerve or muscle weakness, or unexplained confusion. Most neurological care, however, is delivered in outpatient clinics for conditions that can be stabilized and treated routinely, such as migraine headaches, back or neck pain, epilepsy, abnormalities of movement or frequent falls, multiple sclerosis, chronic nerve damage, muscle diseases, memory disorders, and many others.

What Is a Neurosurgeon?

A neurosurgeon is trained in surgical interventions to treat diseases of the brain and spinal cord, and rarely the small nerves of the rest of the body. A neurosurgeon also frequently cares for critically ill patients with brain bleeds, tumors, injuries to the brain or spinal cord, or many other conditions that have new and exciting surgical treatments that never existed before. For example, Parkinson's disease is typically managed with medications, but in some cases a stimulator can be placed by a surgeon in the brain to improve the condition as well. Most neurosurgical care is directed toward deciding if surgery is necessary or not, and if so, a neurosurgeon will follow a patient for the duration of the operative course from planning the surgery to follow-up weeks later. A neurosurgeon will occasionally need to follow a patient in a clinic for years, for example to monitor the stability or growth of aneurysms or tumors.

Who Are Some Other Doctors Who Care for Neurological Patients?

Many patients with neurological disease will also receive care from a doctor with specialty training in physical medicine and rehabilitation (frequently called "PM&R" or physiatry).

A neurologist may help diagnose and prevent a condition such as stroke, but the physiatrist role is to help direct treatment to get the patient better from the condition through medications for muscle relaxation, exercises such as physical therapy, and frequently office procedures for pain control.

Many patients with neurological disorders also have behavioral effects of their disease. As a result, psychiatrists, or mental health doctors, treat patients for depression, anxiety, sleep disorders, aggression, or any other behavioral effect of the disease.

Other Providers

In addition to doctors, in modern healthcare, patients often interact with highly specialized nurse practitioners and physician assistants (NPs or PAs). These individuals have graduate degrees in medical care and spend many years practicing in subspecialty care. Depending on the setting, they may work independently of the physician, in the operating room, as part of a hospital team, or in the office. In addition to their roles in providing direct care, these professionals typically help educate patients on their diseases, and assist the team in understanding all the factors that go into a successful treatment plan.

Many other specialists also care for patients, such as nurses, social workers, pharmacists, and of course other doctors. It can be confusing for a patient to understand all the roles of the team members, but they are all there to help, and are willing to discuss their roles at any time.

Understanding the Nervous System

Entire libraries exist to explain the nervous system, and even all those books represent what amounts to a very incomplete understanding of the brain and nervous system biology. This very brief overview will help set the foundation for understanding the vocabulary doctors and nurses use to discuss neurological diseases. Much more information will follow in this book and can also be found online in many resources.

The brain is the central organ of the nervous system. It is a highly organized network of nerves where signals are received, processed, and sent back out to the body. The outer layer of the brain is the cortex, a word that comes from the Latin, for bark, as in the bark of a tree. The cortex in humans is six cell layers, and is also called the grey matter. The control center, or nucleus, of many nerve cells is in the cortex. This thin layer is responsible for all the complexity, majesty, and mystery of the human condition. It is the origin of our personality and our intellect. It is the place where our language develops and resides for all our life. It is where we process vision, hearing, smell, and taste. It is the place all of our memories are formed, and in some cases the reason they diminish. In short, the cortex is what makes us all different from one another.

Underneath the cortex is the white matter. The white matter is the long strands of the nerve cell body that transmits the signals from the cortex to other parts of the brain and eventually to the body. The white matter is much like train tracks that carry signals from one place to another. Injury to this part of the brain, which occurs in diseases like stroke and multiple sclerosis, can cause obvious weakness, sensory loss, or vision loss, or more subtle problems, such as slowed thinking, impaired memories, and worsening mood.

Deeper in the brain are other centers of control that allow us to do many functions that we never consciously think about. For example, coordinating our movements occurs in the cerebellum, while our gait is smoothed by deep centers called the basal ganglia. Basic reflexes, like moving our eyes when we turn our head, occur in the brainstem, as do many other reflexes, such as blinking, coughing, and most fundamentally breathing.

Some signals enter or leave the brain from specialized organs, like the eyes and ears. Most signals, though, exit below our neck to our body via the spinal cord. The spinal cord is the ultimate expressway for carrying nerve messages to and from the brain. At its widest point, the spinal cord is about the size of a thumb. Like a tree going beneath the soil, as it descends from the brain it gives off roots. These nerve roots exit from the bones of the back and into the structures of the arms, chest, abdomen, pelvis, and legs. Any irritation or injury along this pathway can interrupt the flow of information and cut off the brain from the body, meaning the brain can no longer sense or move the body as it should, and the patient will feel numb, weak, or in pain.

As the nerve roots spread through the body, they become smaller nerves that interface with every organ and every inch of every tissue of our bodies. One important example of this interaction is muscles. As nerves reach muscles they dispense a chemical into the microscopic space between the nerve and the muscle itself. These chemical bundles called neurotransmitters cross the small threshold and bind to receptors on the muscle itself. Once bound, the muscle reacts by shortening, and contracting, or moving. This occurs in the tiniest muscles of our ears to keep our ear drum taut and our hearing keen, in the muscles of our eyes to keep our gaze in the direction we wish, in the muscle of our diaphragm which opens our lungs, and in the largest muscles of our legs to make us move. Diseases that injure the nerves carrying the signals, or in the junction of the nerve and muscle typically cause weakness, which may result in double vision, falls, or even trouble breathing.

Keeping the Nervous System Going

The brain cannot support itself, and yet it is the greediest organ of the body, requiring more metabolic energy than any other organ. Although it accounts for only about 2 % of our body weight, it uses about 20 % of our energy. The energy for the brain comes from oxygen in the blood which originates in the lungs and is pumped from the heart to the brain via four major blood vessels or arteries. The two largest arteries are in the front of the neck, and are called the carotids. They supply about 85 % of the brain's blood supply. The two smaller arteries in the back of the neck are called vertebral arteries and supply the brainstem. Any disease that deprives the brain of blood flow, oxygen, or nutrition will cause potentially irreversible brain damage.

Chapter 3
The Neurosurgery Healthcare Team

Wenya Linda Bi and E. Antonio Chiocca

Introduction

Neurosurgery is comprised of a diverse range of disease conditions involving the brain, spine, peripheral nerves, and blood vessels that supply these vital structures. The care of neurosurgery patients involves an equally complex and mutually integrative group of health care professionals. While each individual serves a slightly different role, effective communication between the team, the patient, and family is crucial to maximizing safe and efficient care.

Team Composition

Your first encounter with the neurosurgery team may be in the emergency room, the clinic, or within the inpatient hospital setting. No matter the location, an integral core of a neurosurgery attending, or the primary physician responsible for the neurosurgical care delivered, occasional residents and fellows, who are physicians undergoing further subspecialty

W.L. Bi, MD, PhD • E.A. Chiocca, MD, PhD (✉)
Department of Neurosurgery, Brigham and Women's Hospital,
15 Francis Street, PBB-3, Boston, MA 02115, USA
e-mail: eachiocca@partners.org

A. Agrawal, G. Britz (eds.), *Comprehensive Guide to Neurosurgical Conditions*, DOI 10.1007/978-3-319-06566-3_3,
© Springer International Publishing Switzerland 2015

training in neurosurgery, nurses, and ancillary support staff exists. Physician's assistants (P.A.s) and nurse practioners (N.P.s) augment the neurosurgical team in many institutions, often offering the initial triage and management of a clinical situation as well as reporting any critical situations to the responding surgeon.

Emergency Encounters

Should your initial encounter be in the emergency room, you may interact with a rapidly changing set of personnel as medical needs are triaged and new diagnostic concerns arise. The emergency department clinician solicits the primary symptoms affecting the patient and orders the initial imaging and laboratory tests. Based on their degree of concern for the problem at hand, they may contact the neurosurgery team immediately or after the initial results return. The first neurosurgical team member to assess the patient may be a resident, fellow, or physician's assistant. This individual will have the clinical experience to make initial recommendations, triage and intervene on emergent situations, and call upon the support of more seasoned neurosurgeons should any questions arise.

Clinic Encounters

Patients, who are deemed to be medically stable but with a neurologic condition that requires follow-up evaluation, may be seen in the clinic, which is also known as the outpatient setting. There, another team of nurses, N.P.s, P.A.s, neurosurgical trainees, and administrative assistants work with the primary neurosurgical attending to provide your care. The nurse, N.P., or P.A. provides continuity of care and may be more readily accessible for routine questions than the neurosurgeon, who may be operating or taking care of other emergencies. A billing manager is available in many practices to help overcome logistical barriers such as insurance and financial concerns. Coordination with other physicians to establish multi-disciplinary appointments within the same trip often happens. When appropriate, patients are referred to neurology, ophthalmology, otolaryngology, oncology, radiation oncology, or neuro-endocrine clinic for further evaluation of a complex problem.

Hospital Settings

If a patient is admitted to the hospital, another wide array of inpatient team members will contribute to the care. Perhaps the most vital figure in day-to-day care is the bedside nurse, who will administer crucial and often complex regimens of medications, monitor for the first sign of worsening neurologic condition, communicate with the physician team any concerns, and support the family and friends in a relatable manner. Multiple times during the day, often early in the morning and then again in the late afternoon or evening, neurosurgeons will come to visit the patient personally, in a process referred to as medical rounds. During these visits, the physician typically performs a brief physical exam to monitor progress of critical symptoms or signs for which the patient is being treated. Discussions about upcoming surgical interventions, the anticipated recovery course, or any questions from the patient and family should be addressed to the physician during rounds. Further check-ups throughout the day depend on the number of active medical issues that need to be resolved, as well as any nursing concerns that arise. Although the supervising neurosurgeon may not be present at bedside as regularly as the rest of the team, rest assured that he or she remains up-to-date on any critical issues and remains the ultimate responsible physician for the patient's care.

The Path to Recovery

Given the nature of neurosurgical diseases, many patients benefit from physical therapy, occupational therapy, speech or swallow evaluations, and nutrition evaluation. Physical therapists assess the safety and mobility of patients as well as provide instruction on how to adapt to and improve upon any disabilities. Occupational therapists assess cognitive impairment, many of which are temporary in the acute post-operative period, and offer adaptive strategies for deficits in visual-spatial attention or perception. Occupational therapists are also especially trained to work with hand and arm weakness or incoordination. Swallow and speech dysfunction is common among the neurosurgical patient population, either due to direct disease infiltration of the regions controlling these functions, or due to prolonged disability from a severely depressed mental state. Specialists routinely perform bedside or formal imaging-guided assessments of swallowing and make recommendations on the risk of choking, also known as aspiration. Sometimes, patients benefit from a temporary feeding tube to provide adequate nutrition, which can be easily removed after improvement in swallowing safety.

If the neurological disability is severe enough to prevent functional adaptability at home, even with support, then the medical team and therapists may recommend a stay at a rehabilitation facility. A care coordinator who has intimate knowledge of the strengths of available regional rehabilitation facilities, as well as how to facilitate transfer to distant facilities that may be more convenient for the patient's family or overall recovery, will become critical at this stage. The care coordinator, often in conjunction with a social worker, can help with insurance and financial concerns as well. Times of critical illness can bring together family, friends, and individuals of disparate paths. Relationship strains may need to be put aside or resolved for the sake of an ill loved one. Issues of guardianship, contacting estranged family members, and other frequently challenging personal conflicts may be assuaged by the social worker.

Maintaining Effective Communication

The inherently busy nature of neurosurgery, with frequent unexpected emergent situations, may appear to divert attention away from routine communication between the surgeon and patients. However, the fundamental network of nurses, residents, fellows, N.P.s, P.A.s, social workers, and other support staff are mutually complementary and exist to eradicate barriers to communication. It is the obligation of the neurosurgical care team to provide timely updates and realistic projections for necessary steps in the care and recovery of the patient. It is equally important for patients and families to voice their questions and concerns in a timely manner to avoid unnecessary miscommunications.

A perfect surgery can only result in the desired clinical outcome with vigilant peri-operative preparation and postoperative care, which requires a team approach. The patient, family, and friend support network are integral players in this team. Ultimately, the clinical staff and all auxiliary services exist to maximize the safety, care, and prognosis of the neurosurgical patient.

Chapter 4
Neurosurgical Intensive Care Unit

Jessica McElheny, Sankalp Gokhale, and David L. McDonagh

Intensive Care to Neurocritical Care

It is difficult to highlight the beginnings of neurocritical care without first discussing the origin of the intensive care unit. Intensive care units or ICU's originated as more invasive and complex treatment options became available for respiratory failure [1]. The instigating event was the polio epidemic in the 1950s. Polio is a viral illness that causes paralysis of many muscle groups including those that are responsible for breathing [2]. During that time the first ventilator known as the Iron Lung (Fig. 4.1) was put into use to support breathing until a recovery could be made [3]. Peter Safar, an Anesthesiologist, is credited with pioneering cardiopulmonary resuscitation (CPR) [4]. He wrote a book

J. McElheny (✉) • S. Gokhale
Departments of Neurology, Duke University Medical Center, Durham, NC, USA
e-mail: jessica.mcelheny@dm.duke.edu

D.L. McDonagh
Departments of Neurology, Duke University Medical Center, Durham, NC, USA

Departments of Anesthesiology, Duke University Medical Center, Durham, NC, USA

A. Agrawal, G. Britz (eds.), *Comprehensive Guide to Neurosurgical Conditions*, DOI 10.1007/978-3-319-06566-3_4, © Springer International Publishing Switzerland 2015

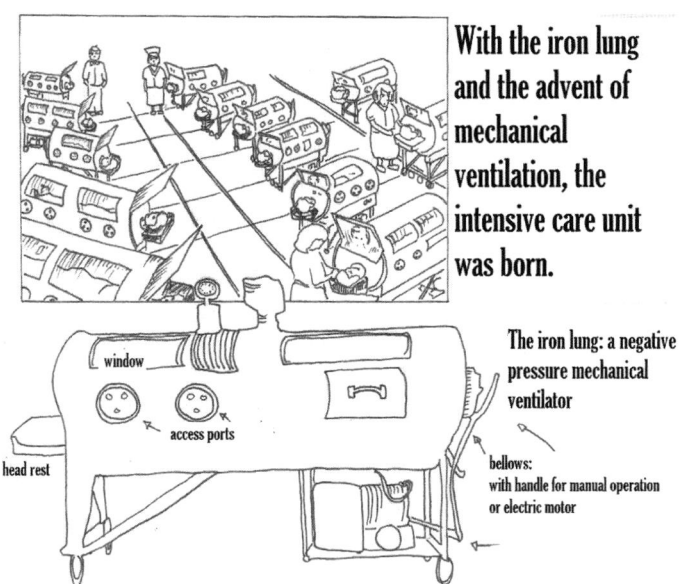

With the iron lung and the advent of mechanical ventilation, the intensive care unit was born.

The iron lung: a negative pressure mechanical ventilator

window

access ports

head rest

bellows: with handle for manual operation or electric motor

FIGURE 4.1 Schematic representation of iron lung. Iron lung was very first form of mechanical ventilator (Breathing machine)

titled "The ABC of Resuscitation" in 1957 for training the public in CPR. He also started the first intensive care unit (ICU) in 1958 in the USA [5].

Since that time, medical and surgical options have continued to progress for conditions that had previously not been survivable. The catch was that patients who formerly would not have survived were in fact alive and they were sicker than ever. This new population of very sick people with very unique and complex illnesses drove the need for dedicated specialty ICU's. For example, a person who had brain surgery yesterday had very different needs than someone who had had a heart attack. Today, most large medical centers have separate ICU's for general and cardiac surgery, general and cardiac medicine, trauma, burn patients, neurology and neurosurgery, and others depending on institutional need.

Dr. Walter Dandy a neurosurgeon at Johns Hopkins Hospital can be credited with championing the neurocritical care movement at Johns Hopkins Hospital in the 1930s [6, 7]. He recognized that neurosurgical patients needed vigilant monitoring during the immediate postoperative period to quickly identify, and treat any complications. At first it was the surgeons who saw their patients in the ICU, but eventually they realized that they could not be present both in the ICU and in the operating room simultaneously and couldn't keep up with the day-to-day demands of patient care in the operating room and neurosurgical ICU [8]. The result was the development of specialty providers to provide this service [9]. These specialists were often anesthesiologists and neurologists with interest and special training in critical care. In time, they brought their respective skills together and formed a uniquely talented team to provide comprehensive care for patients recovering from brain surgery [10] (Table 4.1).

Evolution

Eventually, many neurosurgical intensive care units started to admit patients with non-operative neurologic conditions, such as strokes, seizures, brain hemorrhages, traumatic brain injury, tumors, infections, and spinal cord injuries, as well as diseases of the peripheral neuromuscular system (diseases of the nerves that run from the spinal cord to the muscles or of the muscles themselves) such as myasthenia gravis, and Guillain-Barre. These ICU's eventually began to be known as neuroscience intensive care units or neuro-ICU's in late 1980s & early 1990s [11]. The growing number of patients requiring care in these units prompted the development of physician training programs and societies (ex. The Neurocritical Care Society http://www.neurocriticalcare.org) dedicated to this unique science [12].

The focus of neurocritical care is to treat severe injuries and illnesses of the brain, spinal cord, and peripheral nerves. Injury to the neurologic system is associated with and precipitates a spectrum of dysfunction of other organs. Neurocritical care is aimed at treating and supporting these other organs systems as well. The Neurocritical Care Society

TABLE 4.1 Common terminology used in the neuroscience intensive care unit

Stroke	The word stroke is a catchall term used to describe a brain injury that is caused either by a blockage of blood flow or bleeding into the brain.
Ischemic stroke	An ischemic stroke is when the brain is injured from a lack of blood flow due to a blocked blood vessel in the brain (Similar to a heart attack).
Intracerebral Hemorrhage (ICH)	Intracerebral hemorrhage is a type of stroke that occurs when a blood vessel in the brain bursts and results in a collection of blood in the brain.
Subarachnoid Hemorrhage (SAH)	Subarachnoid hemorrhage is another type of stroke that happens when a weakened blood vessel called an aneurism ruptures and causes bleeding into a part of the brain called the subarachnoid space.
Vasospasm	Vasospasm is a condition associated with SAH (subarachnoid hemorrhage) where the blood vessels in the brain narrow and can limit blood flow to the brain causing ischemic strokes.
Endovascular	Endovascular describes the type of method that is used to repair weakened blood vessels (aneurysms) that can cause subarachnoid hemorrhages. It involves putting a line similar to an IV into the artery in the groin and feeding a wire into the brain to fix the broken blood vessel. The alternative to this is brain surgery to clip the weakened blood vessel.
Seizures	The brain uses tiny electrical signals to send information from one place to another. Seizures occur when many signals fire at the same time, and can cause a person to lose consciousness and or have abnormal jerking of body parts.

TABLE 4.1 (continued)

Hydrocephalus	There are several structures in the brain that are filled with spinal fluid. Under usual circumstances the production and absorption of spinal fluid are equal. Sometimes for various reasons an imbalance happens resulting in excess spinal fluid, which in turn causes increased pressure in the brain. To avoid compressing adjacent parts of the brain, shunts are often placed to drain the fluid.
Cerebrospinal Fluid (CSF)	CSF and spinal fluid are synonymous. CSF is a clear colorless fluid that is present in fluid sacs in the brain. It also circulated around and surrounds the brain and spinal cord.
Lumbar Puncture (LP)	Lumbar puncture is also known as a spinal tap, where a small hollow needle is inserted in between the bones of the lower back in order to obtain a sample of spinal fluid for analysis.
Intracranial Pressure (ICP)	Intracranial pressure is the pressure inside the skull. Under normal circumstances the pressure is less than 15 mmHg. In people whose brain has been injured the pressures are often much higher. Our goal is to keep these pressures as low as possible and can be achieved with medications, drains, and surgery.
Motor	The term motor is synonymous with movement and is measured by testing how strong a person is. Damage to different parts of the brain can produce weaknesses of different muscles.
Sensory	Sensory is a word used to describe sensation or feeling. Damage to some parts of the brain can cause numbness or decreased sensation.

(continued)

Table 4.1 (continued)

Meningitis	Meningitis is an infection of the lining of the brain, and is usually tested for by performing a spinal tap.
EEG (electroencephalogram)	EEG is brain wave monitoring that looks for seizures. Small sticky "leads" or stickers are placed on the scalp and detect electrical currents on the surface of the brain. EEG monitoring is analogous to the EKG of heart rhythm monitoring.
GCS (Glasgow Coma Scale)	GCS is a scale that uses a 15 point system to measure of level of consciousness where 15 is a perfect score, less than 8 would be coma, and 3 would be deep coma. Repeat measurements allow caregivers to see how a person is doing over a period of time.
Coma	Coma is a general term used to describe a state of unconsciousness defined by the lack of response to stimuli. (Stimuli can be verbal cues or pain)
Ventilator	A ventilator or respirator is a device used to deliver air and or oxygen to the lungs by way of a tube inserted through the mouth or neck.
Endotracheal Tube (ETT)	An endotracheal tube or ETT is a hollow plastic tube that is placed through a person's mouth and into their lungs. It is used together with a ventilator to provide a clear passage of air flow into the lungs.
External ventricular drain (EVD)	The EVD is a small tube placed into the fluid filled spaces in the brain and can be used to drain excess fluid (CSF) and measure intracranial pressures (ICP)

was founded in 2002 in San Francisco, CA. There are approximately 70–80 dedicated Neuro-ICU's in the United States and the field is progressively expanding [13]. In 2006, the United Council of Neurologic Subspecialties created a credentialing (i.e., certification) pathway for Neurocritical Care Physicians and training requirements (i.e., accreditation) for neurocritical care fellowships [12].

"The Care Team"

Neurointensivists are physicians who have trained in neurology, anesthesiology, or emergency medicine (i.e. Completed residency) and who have completed a 2 year fellowship in neurocritical care. Neurosurgeons also participate in neurocritical care and some work in part as neurointensivists. Acute Care Nurse Practitioners (ACNP's), Pharmacists, Critical Care certified Registered Nurses (CCRN's), Respiratory Therapists (RT's), Nutritionists, Physical and Occupational therapists, Speech Therapists, Social workers and Pastoral Services form a comprehensive team of trained professionals dedicated to taking care of patients in the neurocritical care unit. Clinical data has shown that patients with acute nervous system injury do much better when admitted to specialized neurocritical care units as compared to general critical care units [14].

Brain Matters

The brain requires special consideration because it is absolutely essential to functioning as a living organism. The brain is the control center for all of the body's functions. It provides thought, movement, sensation, walking, talking, swallowing, hearing, tasting, and seeing, just to name a few functions. It has several main parts including the cerebrum,

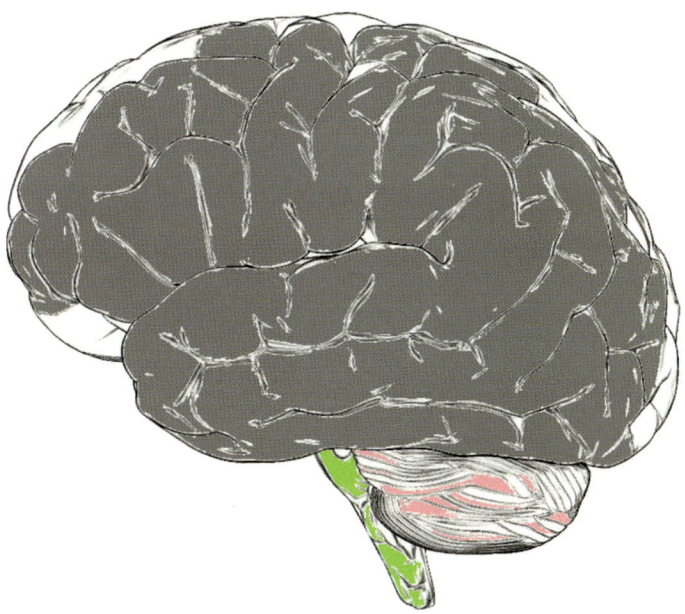

FIGURE 4.2 Schematic representation of human brain showing major parts. Cerebrum (colored in *grey*), cerebellum (*pink*) and brainstem (*green*)

cerebellum, and brainstem (Fig. 4.2). The cerebrum is what makes us who we are. It is the part of the brain that is concerned with personality, planning, speech, movement, and the perception of sight, sound, and touch. The cerebellum deals with muscle coordination and balance, while the brainstem controls breathing, heart rate, blood pressure, swallowing, and speaking. Temperature, appetite, and thirst are controlled by an area above the brainstem, called the diencephalon (hypothalamus & thalamus). The brainstem leaves the skull to become the spinal cord. The spinal cord carries signals for movement and sensation (touch, feeling) from the brain to the body and vice versa. The left side of the brain controls the right side of the body and vice versa, so damage to the right side of the brain produces problems with the left side of the body. This is even true for vision, where the left side of the brain sees the right side of things we see, and vice versa.

The brain and spinal cord are encased in bone to protect them from physical harm. The skull is a bony vault that encases the brain and is met at its base by the bones of the neck, which are also known as vertebrae, and is where the spinal cord exits the skull. The vertebrae cover and protect the spinal cord and form what we know as 'the spine'.

When the brain is injured whether it is from bleeding, stroke, or trauma, it has a tendency to swell like any other injured part of the body. Imagine for a moment, hitting your thumb with a hammer. It would become red and swollen to facilitate healing. The rigid skull, although it works well to protect the brain from trauma does not allow for swelling. The result of this is increased pressures inside the skull that are then applied to the brain tissue. These increased pressures can compress and damage brain tissue that had not previously been injured. This concept is important to understand because many of our interventions in the neuroscience ICU are aimed at reducing the brain pressure while maximizing the delivery of blood and oxygen. For example, many patients require removal of fluid from within the brain or even removal of part of the skull to reduce pressure in the skull after huge strokes or after traumatic brain injury.

Some of the necessity of having a special ICU devoted to neurological conditions is expertise and use of brain monitoring devices. These devices are placed either into the brain tissue itself, or into the fluid filled spaces in the brain known as the ventricles. These monitors are used in conjunction with frequent neurologic examinations to see how a person is responding to changing variables. Other special monitoring devices include continuous brain wave monitoring (called EEG or electroencephalography) which is used to look for seizure activity (Fig. 4.3).

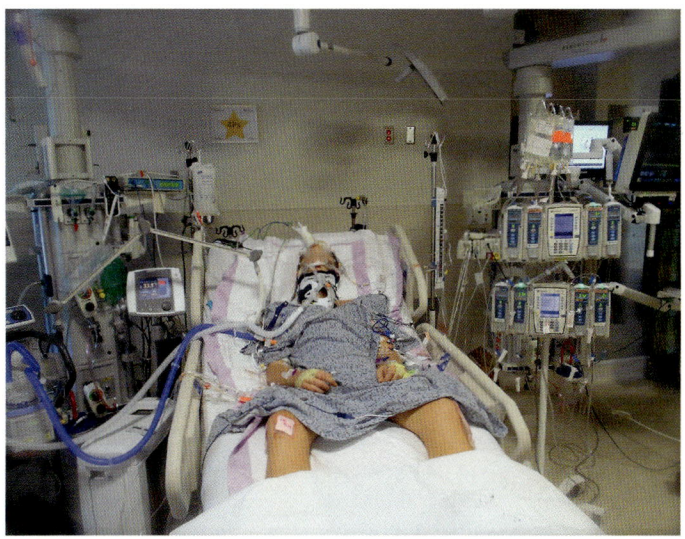

FIGURE 4.3 Modern day neurocritical care unit. Complex multi-modal neuromonitring allows for accurate and detailed assessment of critically sick patients and allows for quick and effective treatment strategies

A Day in the Life

Life in the neurocritical care unit revolves around frequent, often hourly neurologic examinations, heart and respiratory function monitoring, diagnostic testing and treatment. It can be exhausting both for patients and their loved ones as well. We understand that this is a difficult time and try our best to facilitate a restful environment between interventions.

The physicians directing the care of your loved one most often are neurointensivists, neurologists, or neurosurgeons. They work closely with nurse practitioners, physician assistants, resident physicians, respiratory therapists, and pharmacists. These health care professionals will visit your loved one at least once or more often each day. Other things to expect include daily and often more frequent blood draws, physical, occupational, and speech therapy sessions, medications, CT and MRI scans, and brainwave monitoring. For the sickest patients artificial breathing support may be necessary to ensure adequate lung function. Most cases involve a breathing tube (endotracheal tube or ETT) that is placed into the lungs. The end of the tube that comes out of the mouth is then connected to the respirator (or ventilator). Being on a respirator often causes some degree of discomfort; to ameliorate this, patients are kept on sedating medications to keep them comfortable. In these instances it is paramount to balance the need for sedation with the ability to conduct neurologic examinations.

In addition, procedures may be performed to improve or enhance care. Some of these include the placement of central lines to administer intravenous medications, arterial lines to continuously monitor blood pressure, feeding tubes to provide early nutrition, and drains to empty urine from the bladder. Tubes called external ventricular drains or EVD's may be placed into the brain to monitor brain pressures and drain spinal fluid if necessary. Patients requiring ventilator support for many days may need a tracheostomy (surgery on the neck to insert a breathing tube). Similarly, patients who cannot swallow may need a nasogastric tube, going through the nose into the stomach, or a semi-permanent gastrostomy tube (aka, 'PEG') that goes under the rib cage directly into the stomach.

It would be a great disservice if I did not mention the importance of the bedside nurse in caring for the neurocritical care patient. Neurocritical care nurses have specialty training to care for both severe neurologic illness but also the frequently occurring dysfunction in other organ systems. Their specialty training and presence at the bedside improves communication between the rest of the critical care team and the patient/family. This expertise also allows for the early identification and intervention of complications. They are the guardian angels for the neurocritical care patient.

The Future

One of the many benefits of large academic medical centers and specialty intensive care units is that they often serve as a hub for research. At any given time at our institution we may have up to six or seven separate studies enrolling patients. This research is of the utmost importance for gathering information about how we can improve the care and treatments offered to patients with severe neurologic illnesses. In the meantime, we continue to work diligently at the bedside to provide quality, evidenced-based care to those patients and families who presently occupy our neuroscience intensive care units.

References

1. Hilberman M. The evolution of intensive care units. Crit Care Med. 1975;3(4):159–65.
2. Nathanson N, Kew OM. From emergence to eradication: the epidemiology of poliomyelitis deconstructed. Am J Epidemiol. 2010;172(11):1213–29.
3. Lassen HC. A preliminary report on the 1952 epidemic of poliomyelitis in Copenhagen with special reference to the treatment of acute respiratory insufficiency. Lancet. 1953;1(6749):37–41.
4. Weil MH, Shoemaker WC. Pioneering contributions of Peter Safar to intensive care and the founding of the Society of Critical Care Medicine. Crit Care Med. 2004;32(2 Suppl):S8–10.
5. Rosengart MR. Critical care medicine: landmarks and legends. Surg Clin North Am. 2006;86(6):1305–21.
6. Bleck TP. Historical aspects of critical care and the nervous system. Crit Care Clin. 2009;25(1):153–64, ix.
7. Pearce JM. Walter Edward Dandy (1886–1946). J Med Biogr. 2006;14(3):127–8.
8. Wijdicks EF, Worden WR, Miers A, Piepgras DG. The early days of the neurosciences intensive care unit. Mayo Clin Proc. 2011;86(9):903–6.
9. Long DM. A century of change in neurosurgery at Johns Hopkins: 1889–1989. J Neurosurg. 1989;71(5 Pt 1):635–8.

10. Ropper AH. Neurological intensive care. Ann Neurol. 1992;32(4):564–9.
11. Rincon F, Mayer SA. Neurocritical care: a distinct discipline? Curr Opin Crit Care. 2007;13(2):115–21.
12. Mayer SA, Coplin WM, Chang C, et al. Core curriculum and competencies for advanced training in neurological intensive care: United Council for Neurologic Subspecialties guidelines. Neurocrit Care. 2006;5(2):159–65.
13. Ward MJ, Shutter LA, Branas CC, Adeoye O, Albright KC, Carr BG. Geographic access to US Neurocritical Care Units registered with the Neurocritical Care Society. Neurocrit Care. 2012;16(2):232–40.
14. Suarez JI, Zaidat OO, Suri MF, et al. Length of stay and mortality in neurocritically ill patients: impact of a specialized neurocritical care team. Crit Care Med. 2004;32(11):2311–7.

Chapter 5
Common Neuroradiological Procedures

Leo Galvin, Katherine E. Wood, and David S. Enterline

Introduction

An important aspect in the evaluation and treatment of most medical conditions is imaging, or taking a picture of the inside of the body using a machine. Radiology is a medical specialty whose doctors have special training in the imaging of all parts of the human body. Radiologists work with other physicians to diagnose and treat patients by using a broad arsenal of sophisticated technologies, such as computed tomography (CT) and magnetic resonance imaging (MRI). These tools are routinely used to diagnose a wide variety of medical and surgical conditions. Additionally, radiologists can use imaging to help guide procedures. These procedures can include biopsy and drainage, placement of central catheters and ports, and diagnosis and therapy with angiography.

A neuroradiologist is a doctor who is trained and specialized in radiology with additional training and expertise in imaging and image-guided treatment of disorders of the central nervous system (CNS), including the brain and spine. Neuroradiologists work closely with neurosurgeons.

L. Galvin, MD, MRCPI, FFRRCSI • D.S. Enterline (✉), MD, FACR
Department of Radiology, Duke University, Durham, NC
e-mail: david.enterline@duke.edu

K.E. Wood, BS
Houston Methodist, Houston, TX

A. Agrawal, G. Britz (eds.), *Comprehensive Guide to Neurosurgical Conditions*, DOI 10.1007/978-3-319-06566-3_5,
© Springer International Publishing Switzerland 2015

When the results of a scan are given to a patient, the formal report will have been issued by a neuroradiologist. Often the imaging results will have been discussed directly between the neurosurgeon and neuroradiologist. The field of neuroscience has advanced in recent decades at an incredible rate- as neurosurgical techniques evolve and become more sophisticated so too does neuroradiology. The strong collaboration between these two specialties continues to result in more accurate and timely diagnosis and ultimately more successful management of even the most complex diseases of the brain and spine, including cancer.

This chapter outlines the most common imaging procedures likely to be encountered by a patient with a neurosurgical disorder. In each section we will offer a brief background on a specific technology, what to expect if you are having this test, and discuss how it might provide imaging findings to diagnose common neurosurgical disorders of the brain and spine. These findings and diagnoses contribute to overall patient care and can result in better outcomes. It is our goal to educate patients and their families about these common imaging procedures and interventions. In doing so we hope that they feel well informed and less anxious when seeking and undergoing examinations and procedures for a wide variety of neurological disorders.

Plain Radiography (X-ray)

What Is It?

Radiographs are obtained by using x-rays to obtain a 2D image of the body. Formerly, this was a photographic type film but now is almost exclusively a digital picture format. Differences in tissue density interacting with ionizing x-rays provide the radiographical image. The more dense a structure, the better it shows up on the image. For example, bone is dense and is well seen. Plain radiography plays a valuable role in imaging of the spine, particularly in cases of trauma or arthritis. The radiologist evaluates alignment of the bones, fractures, and reactive changes due to various disease processes or injuries. Devices in the body can be seen including shunt catheters and valve settings, and metallic hardware in the spine (Fig. 5.1).

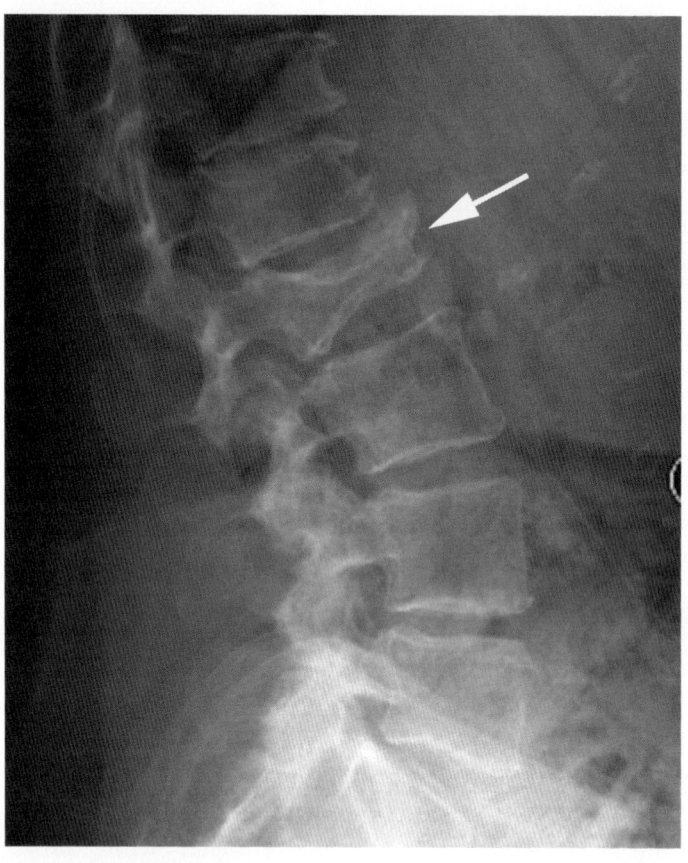

FIGURE 5.1 Plain radiograph of the lumbar spine, lateral projection. There is a chronic fracture of the second lumbar vertebral body (*arrow*). The vertebra has been compressed and has lost significant height with mild forward angulation of the spinal column (kyphosis) at this level

What Does the Procedure Entail?

The patient is placed in either the standing or lying position. Then an x-ray tube is positioned over the relevant body part and a quick snapshot is taken. Multiple views may be needed. This painless procedure is over quickly.

Computed Tomography (CT)

What Is It?

CT is a sophisticated piece of x-ray based equipment that obtains a cross-sectional visualization of the body. It plays a central role in the workup and management of neurological disease. Similar to plain radiography, CT uses x-rays that are carefully controlled and monitored. A rotating x-ray tube and detector array combines with a complex computer to create images that represent those structures being imaged. The images produced are sequential layers or slices of the area of interest. The scans are quick to perform in most cases.

What Does the Procedure Entail?

The patient lies on a table that moves part or all of the body into the center of the scanner, which looks like a giant doughnut. Patients are sometimes given a special contrast agent into a vein, depending on the needs of the study.

CT of the Brain

The most common use of CT in neuroradiology is imaging of the brain. CT is particularly helpful in detecting acute intra-cranial hemorrhage (bleeding), contusions (bruising), stroke, edema (swelling) and hydrocephalus (enlargement of the normal spaces that contain cerebrospinal fluid). CT can also be useful in evaluating certain brain tumors, particularly in patients who cannot have an MRI (Fig. 5.2).

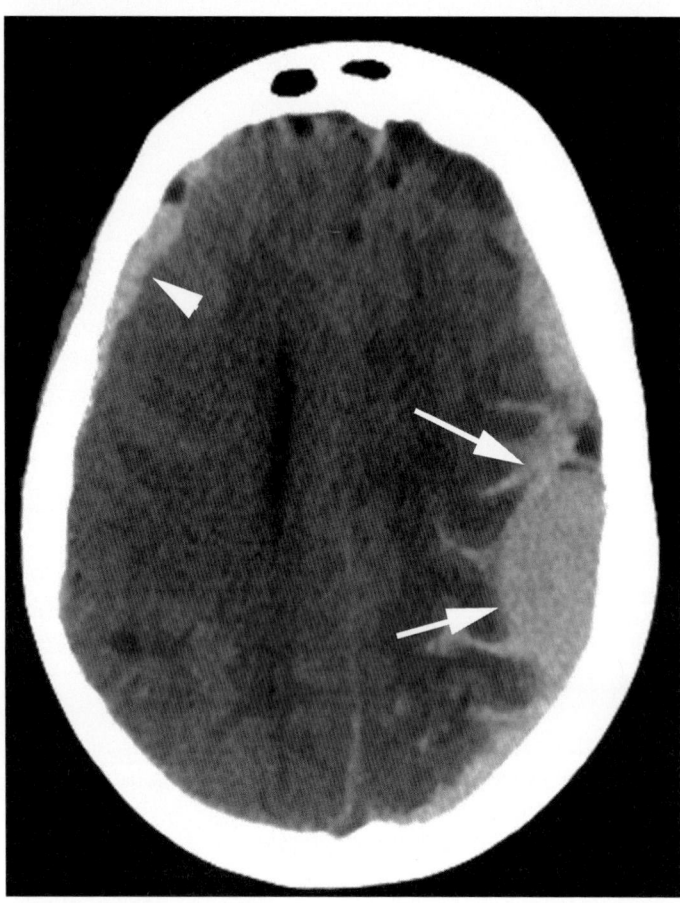

FIGURE 5.2 CT of the brain. There is acute hemorrhage (*white*) overlying the left (*arrows*) and to a lesser extent the right (*arrowhead*) sides of the brain. This patient was involved in a high velocity motor vehicle accident. The head CT, performed shortly after arrival in the emergency room, facilitated rapid diagnosis and subsequent emergent life-saving neurosurgical evacuation of the larger left-sided brain hemorrhage

CT Angiography (CTA)

CT angiography is the term used to describe the imaging of arteries (CT arteriography) and/or veins (CT venography). CTA enables neuroradiologists to view the blood vessels of the head without the surrounding brain tissue or skull. First, a patient is given a contrast agent that makes the blood vessels visible. A CT scan is then performed with sub-millimeter thin images. Finally, computer modeling is used to see the blood vessels. This method has revolutionized the diagnosis of ruptured brain aneurysms and other abnormalities of blood vessels such as arteriovenous malformations (AVMs) (Fig. 5.3).

CT Perfusion (CTP)

This technique measures blood flow to the brain and offers an indirect assessment of blood volume, flow, and transit through the region of imaged brain. A contrast agent is administered and the brain is rapidly imaged to understand how blood moves through brain tissue. It can help characterize certain brain tumors but is more commonly used in the assessment of acute stroke by identifying damaged but still salvageable portions of the brain.

CT of the Spine

CT scans of the spine are typically done in segments of the body: cervical (neck region), thoracic (chest region), or lumbar (abdominal region). Cross-sectional images are viewed separately and can be combined or reformatted with others in different planes to see alignment of the spine. Because of its strength in the assessment of bony structures compared with soft tissues such as ligaments and muscles, CT is the gold standard in the initial imaging of serious spinal trauma. It also provides excellent evaluation of degenerative changes of arthritis and positioning of surgically placed metal screws and cages following spine surgery.

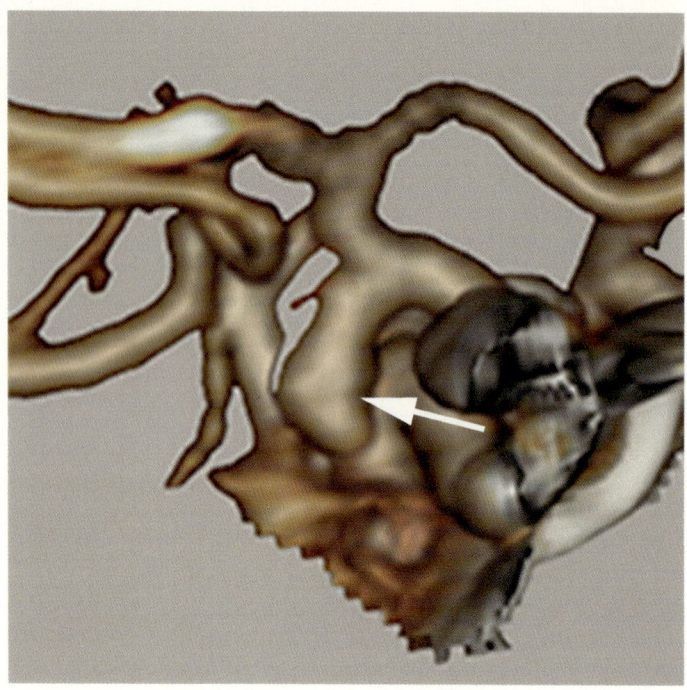

FIGURE 5.3 CT angiography of the brain with 3D reconstruction image. A patient admitted with sudden acute life-threatening brain hemorrhage was found to have a ruptured 7 mm brain aneurysm arising from the distal right carotid artery (*arrow*). The patient was brought to the operating room that night for aneurysm repair and made a full recovery

CT-guided Intervention

CT scans can be performed prior to surgery or during a procedure to improve localizing an area of interest. If the scan is going to be used during surgery, the data is sent to the operating room and used for operative planning. Like a GPS roadmap, the surgeon can view the images and use that data to guide his/her instruments with more precision. Another helpful use of CT is to assist the placement of small needles used for biopsies to obtain tissue or injection of steroid in the management of chronic back pain with or without radiculopathy, the medical term for what is commonly known as "sciatica". The CT-guided images allow for high accuracy during these types of procedures.

Magnetic Resonance Imaging (MRI)

What Is It?

MRI has been widely used since the 1980s and has significantly improved since that time. MRI is particularly useful in imaging disorders of the brain and spinal cord. MRI works by positioning the patient in a very strong magnetic field and then using radio waves which are received by detectors. Complex computer analysis then determines the different anatomic and chemical structures of the tissues being imaged. These result in exquisite detail with better resolution of soft tissues, including the brain, compared to any other radiological modality. One of the advantages is that MRI does not use ionizing radiation. A disadvantage is that MRI may be contraindicated in individuals with certain implantable metallic devices, including most cardiac pacemakers and neurostimulators. If you have metal in your body, it is important to tell the MR technologist before entering the magnet area.

What Does the Procedure Entail?

You lie on a table that moves part or all of your body into the center of the scanner. The middle opening or bore of an MRI machine is smaller than the CT machine, but can vary with the specific machine used. A fan blows cool air over top of the patient. It is noisy during the exam and ear plugs or headphones with music are given. Some individuals with claustrophobia may need mild anti-anxiety (relaxant) medications to help make the experience more comfortable. Make sure to leave your belongings outside the scanning room as the magnetic field around the MRI machine may damage them. Depending on the type of study ordered and indication (what is being evaluated), MRI scans may be done after giving a patient an intravenous contrast agent. This medication is different than the contrast agent used in CT. Your kidney function may be checked prior to the exam if a contrast agent is going to be used.

MRI of the Brain and Spine

MRI offers superior contrast resolution of soft tissues making it possible to distinguish one soft tissue from another. It is the most sensitive and specific test for many diseases. This makes MRI very valuable in the evaluation of CNS infections, inflammatory diseases, stroke, tumors, and many other conditions. The superior contrast resolution of MRI over CT also enables neuroradiologists to appreciate more clearly the soft tissues of the spinal column. In the spine, paraspinal muscles and ligaments, the spinal cord and nerve roots, and disc disease are readily visualized with MRI (Figs. 5.4 and 5.5).

MR Arteriography (MRA) and MR Venography (MRV)

This technique involves the imaging of the arteries and/or veins within the brain. Unlike CT angiography, MRI can use special techniques and blood flow alone in a vessel to create an image. MRA is used to evaluate vascular disorders of the brain, neck, and spine, such as vessel narrowing and blockages, aneurysms and AVMs.

MR Perfusion (MRP)

The MR perfusion technique measures blood flow to the brain and is used predominantly for imaging brain tumors

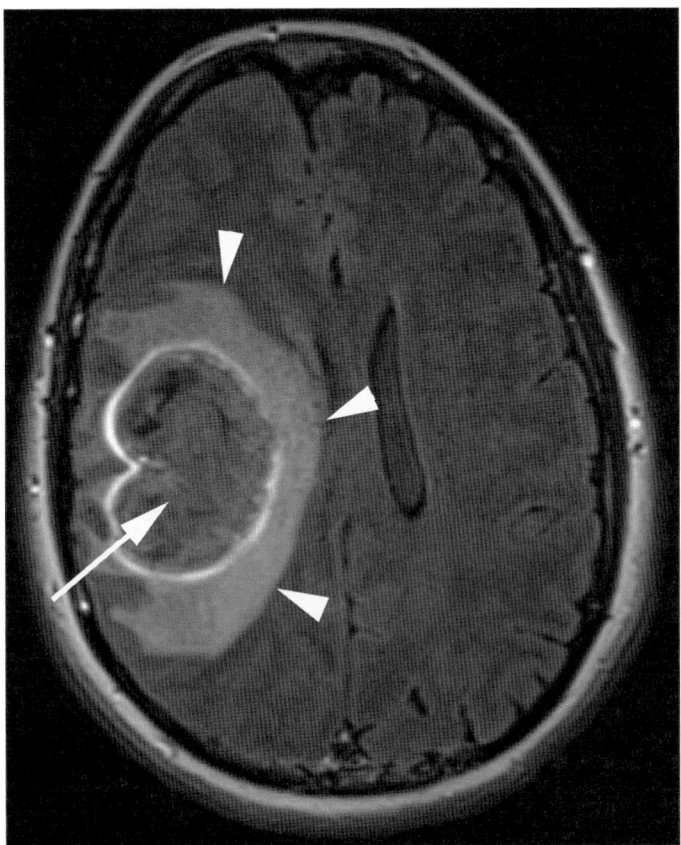

FIGURE 5.4 MRI of the brain. This image demonstrates a large malignant brain tumor (*arrow*). The surrounding grayish halo of swelling (*arrowheads*) gives a clue to the aggressive nature of this particular tumor

and stroke. There has been much research in recent years focusing on MRP in brain tumors since it can provide helpful information on the potential for aggressive tumor behavior (tumor grade).

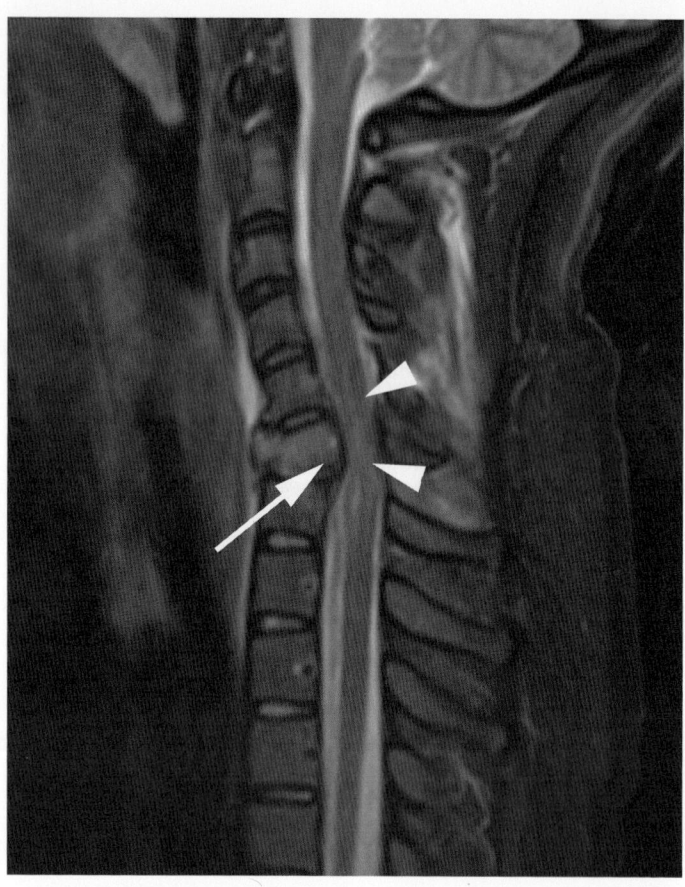

FIGURE 5.5 MRI of the cervical spine. This young patient dived into shallow water and fractured the sixth cervical vertebral body (*arrow*). There is significant resultant narrowing of the spinal canal and severe compression of the spinal cord (*arrowheads*), unfortunately resulting in quadriplegia

Functional MRI (fMRI)

Traditional imaging techniques such as standard MRI and CT evaluate size, shape, structure, substance and other physical qualities of tissue (anatomical data). fMRI offers an added feature and gathers functional data: what area of the brain does a particular function, where do the nerves go, and how close is important function to an abnormality such as a brain tumor. fMRI is performed while the patient carries out specific tasks such as speech or hand movement. This advanced technique can identify small critical areas of brain such as a patient's main speech center. This functional data then becomes invaluable information for the neurosurgeon in terms of his/her approach to an operation involving that part of the brain (Fig. 5.6).

MR Spectroscopy (MRS)

This technique aims, at the atomic level, to detect the presence and measure concentration of metabolites in certain tissue. While not in routine use, it can occasionally assist the reporting neuroradiologist in establishing tumor grade and sometimes help differentiate one type of tumor from another or other CNS disorders.

---→

FIGURE 5.6 (**a**). MRI of the brain following intravenous contrast. There is an aggressive tumor in the right cerebral hemisphere (*arrow*). The contrast causes the rim of the tumor to enhance and appear bright. (**b**) Diffusion Tensor Image ("DTI") of the brain. Sometimes referred to as tractography, this is a functional MRI technique that images concentrated bundles of nerve fibers travelling within the brain and to and from the spinal cord. This image demonstrates the main nerve tracts (*arrows*) extending from the top of the brain (removed for clarification) inferiorly towards the brainstem and spinal cord

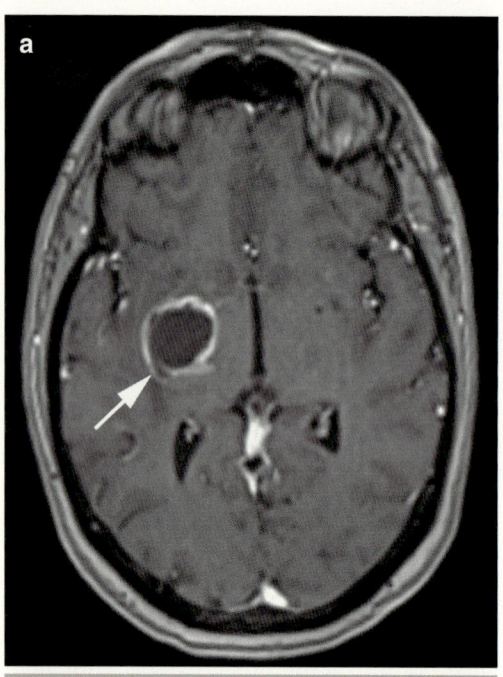

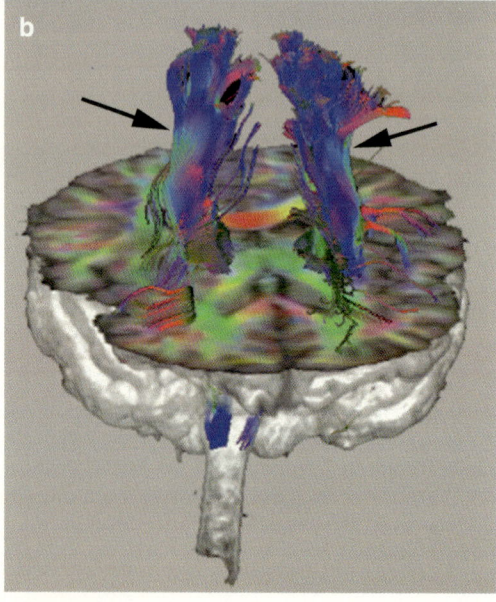

Myelography

What Is It?

Myelography is a test to image the spinal cord and nerve roots within the spinal canal using the injection of a contrast agent into the spinal fluid. Myelograms look for an impression on these structures by bone spurs, herniated disc material, ligaments, and tumor. It can be performed using multiple modalities but usually is done with plain spine radiography followed by spine CT. The contrast agent is well seen on CT and visualizes the adjacent structures. If the myelographic contrast agent is positioned into the head, the procedure is called a cisternogram; this is done to look for cerebrospinal fluid (CSF) leaks (Fig. 5.7).

What Does the Procedure Entail?

For a myelogram, the patient lies on their stomach and a contrast agent is sterilely injected into the thecal sac (the spinal fluid-containing space in the spinal canal). The surrounding skin is numbed so that this causes minimal or no discomfort. An x-ray machine, usually a c-arm, allows the radiologist performing the myelogram under fluoroscopy to see the adjacent bony anatomy for precise needle placement. The technique is similar to performing a lumbar puncture, epidural anesthetic, or epidural steroid injection. A small amount of contrast is injected into the spinal fluid and the table may be tilted to optimally position the contrast agent. X-ray pictures (radiographs) are taken, followed by a CT of the area of interest. Patients may be required to discontinue certain regular medications, such as warfarin, for a few days before the procedure. Your nurse or doctor will tell you about any requirements prior to this procedure.

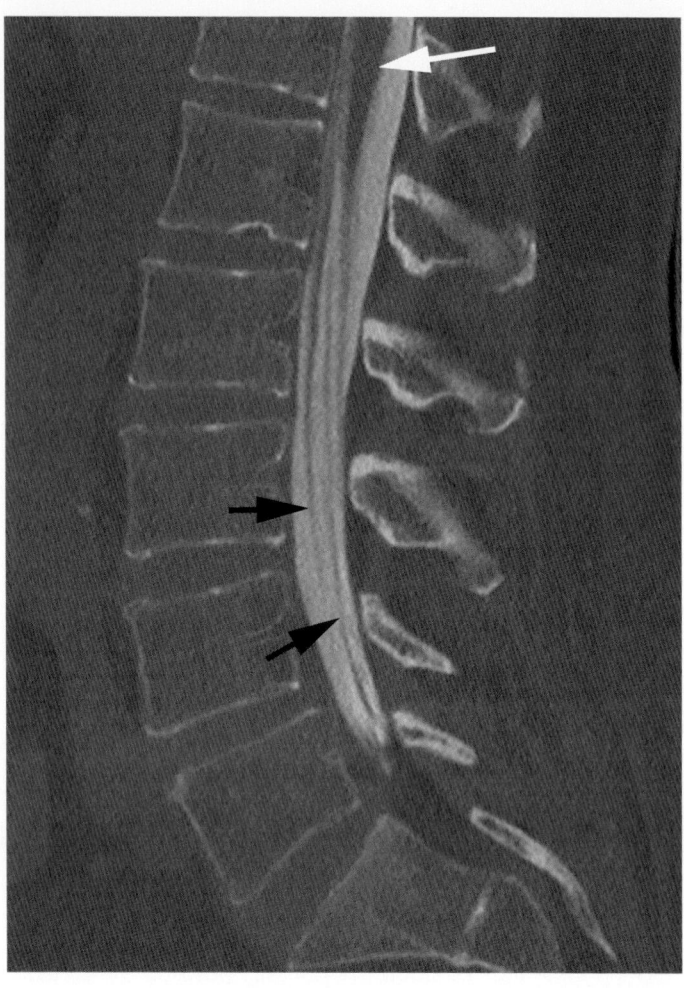

FIGURE 5.7 CT myelogram of the lumbar spine. Contrast has been injected into the spinal fluid causing it to appear bright. The spinal fluid surrounds structures within the spinal canal enabling visualization of the darker appearing spinal cord (*white arrow*) and descending nerve roots (*black arrows*)

Vertebroplasty/Kyphoplasty

What Is It?

Certain conditions can predispose patients to fracture of the vertebral bodies within the spinal column. These fractures can be extremely painful and may heal slowly or not at all. The most common risk factor for a vertebral body fracture is osteoporosis. Vertebroplasty is a minimally invasive procedure that involves injecting a "bone cement" mixture into the fractured vertebral spine bone to fuse the fragments, strengthen the vertebral body and provide pain relief. Kyphoplasty is a similar procedure that creates a small cavity to help direct the cement flow. It also is very effective in eliminating or reducing pain.

What Does the Procedure Entail?

Patients are positioned on their stomach. Moderate sedation for pain relief is administered, as well as local anesthetic at the site of the procedure. Under sterile technique, a needle is then carefully advanced near the front of the broken vertebra. In vertebroplasty, a special cement mixture is injected into the vertebral body. In kyphoplasty, a special balloon or curved needle is used to create a cavity. Special cement is used to fill the cavity created and provide strength to the bone. The procedure typically takes less than 1 h, and is usually performed on an outpatient basis.

Carotid Ultrasound

What Is It?

Abnormal narrowing, known as stenosis, can form due to atherosclerosis ("hardening of the arteries") in one or both of the carotid arteries in the neck. This is a significant risk factor for stroke. There is strong evidence that when carotid artery stenosis reaches a severe degree, reopening the vessel with surgery or an endovascular technique (balloon angioplasty and/or stenting) offers better protection than by medical treatment alone. Carotid ultrasound or sonography evaluates the carotid and vertebral arteries by passing high frequency sound waves from a probe on the skin into the body part of a patient being imaging. The sound waves are reflected back to the probe and an attached computer calculates the depth of the various structures being imaged, permitting an image to be made. The direction and speed of blood flow in a vessel can also be determined using the Doppler Effect. Ultrasound exams are commonly performed to evaluate carotid stenosis and therefore an important tool in the overall workup of stroke.

What Does the Procedure Involve?

A small amount of gel is applied to the skin and an ultrasound probe is gently placed over the neck. The procedure can take anywhere from 10 to 30 min to perform.

Transcranial Doppler (TCD)

What Is It?

This is an ultrasound technique, similar to the description above, except that it focuses on the major arteries of the brain. It is usually performed on critical patients in an intensive care environment. Its main use is to assess inflammatory narrowing of intracranial vessels, known as vasospasm, which is commonly seen in the days and weeks following brain hemorrhage from ruptured intracranial aneurysms.

50 L. Galvin et al.

What Does the Procedure Entail?

A small amount of gel is applied to the temple, just above the ear, and an ultrasound probe is placed over the area. Blood flow velocities are recorded and evaluated.

Suggested Reading

1. American College of Radiology. Radiation safety. http://www.acr.org/Quality-Safety/Radiology-Safety/Radiation-Safety. Accessed July 2014.
2. Castillo M. (2011). Neuroradiology companion: methods, guidelines, and imaging fundamentals. 4th ed. Philadelphia: Lippincott Williams & Wilkins.
3. Huda W. (2009). Review of radiologic physics. 3rd ed. Philadelphia: Lippincott Williams & Wilkins.
4. Osborn AG. (2012). Osborn's brain: imaging, pathology, and anatomy. Philadelphia: Lippincott Williams & Wilkins.
5. Yousem DM, Zimmerman RD, Grossman RI. (2010). Neuroradiology: the requisites. 3rd ed. Missouri: Mosby.

Chapter 6
The Pre-operative and Peri-operative Period

Kristin Lewis and Kai Frerichs

Preoperative

The pre-operative period of surgery is considered to be the time just prior to a surgical procedure beginning when the first preparations take place. Depending on the urgency of the surgery, much of the desired preparation may turn into an unrealistic luxury. Neurological emergencies cross a wide diapason. It is important that quick and appropriate assessments are made with thorough neurological evaluation, as many of these conditions require expeditious initiation of treatment [1].

During this pre-operative time, the focus from the health care team is centered around learning the patient, assessing the patient and educating the patient and family. It is important to learn the patient's nutritional state, medical, surgical and social history, allergies, current medications, and personal habits that may affect his/her health and recovery. It is equally important to assess the patient's physical state, noting any handicaps and/or abnormality, signs of infection, overall general health and appearance, mental state, blood pressure,

K. Lewis, NP (✉) • K. Frerichs, MD
Department of Neurosurgery, Brigham and Women's Hospital,
Boston, MA 02115, USA
e-mail: Klewis1@partners.org

A. Agrawal, G. Britz (eds.), *Comprehensive Guide to Neurosurgical Conditions*, DOI 10.1007/978-3-319-06566-3_6,
© Springer International Publishing Switzerland 2015

heart rate, height and weight. Blood and urine may be taken to check specific lab tests. In case a blood transfusion is necessary during or after the procedure, the patient's blood type will be checked. Often a chest X-ray, electrocardiogram, X-ray, CT and/or MRI scans of the head, neck or spine may be needed. Due to the nature of neurosurgical conditions, a lumbar puncture to check spinal fluid may be necessary.

The patient's and his/her family's understanding of the neurosurgical condition, possible treatments, potential outcomes and prognosis is ascertained. Each of the above is explained in a timely manner to expedite treatment. Oftentimes, the patient is unable to participate in his/her decision-making requiring a family member to be responsible for making decisions and signing consent forms for treatment.

If time permits the patient will need to fast for a short period prior to surgery, typically beginning at midnight the night before. An intravenous will be required to provide fluid during this time if the patient is an inpatient. A bowel preparation may be necessary, as well. Prior to surgery, specific areas of the patient's body will be cleansed with an antibacterial soap. Intravenous access will be gained, which will allow for medications to be given and blood to be drawn quickly and easily. Most likely, a urinary catheter will be placed, and/or a nasogastric tube may be needed, though they are often placed with the patient under sedation or anesthesia for elective procedures.

When patients and families are carefully explained the nature of the condition, planned procedure and potential outcomes, less anxiety is encountered. Family's knowledge of the patient can save a tremendous amount of time, allowing the provider to assess the patient using brief exams.

Perioperative

The perioperative period of surgery begins from the start of surgery until the day of discharge. It is during this period that care, concerns and treatment becomes more focused on the underlying condition. As each individual situation dictates, knowing what to watch for can help identify neurological/post-operative complications, which may require immediate attention.

The brain and spinal cord are complex, each sustained by a system of checks and balances. If one part becomes disrupted or injured, a cascade of complications may ensue. It is important to understand the difference between the primary injury and a secondary injury. The primary injury is that which occurs at the time of insult. The secondary injury is the effects from the initial insult that may compromise other organs, tissue or general perfusion of the cells.

Common Conditions

Ruptured Cerebral Aneurysms/Cerebrovascular Injury

A ruptured aneurysm constitutes a medical emergency due to the potential for life threatening increases in intracranial pressure. If a patient is somnolent or confused, a neurosurgeon will emergently place an external drain to relieve the intracranial pressure—a life saving procedure. Thereafter, the main focus is to secure the ruptured aneurysm to prevent re-rupture and minimize secondary injury to the brain [2]. A ruptured aneurysm may be repaired either by an endovascular approach, inserting and filling the aneurysm with small platinum coils or by open surgery, inserting a metal clip across the base of the aneurysm to prevent flow into the aneurysm. Regardless of which procedure is undertaken, the post-operative period is with similar concerns. Either procedure presents a risk of stroke to the patient—all are thus monitored neurologically in an ICU setting after treatment. A common delayed complication after aneurysm rupture is vasospasm of the blood vessels, whereby the vessels narrow (spasm) causing decreased blood flow, putting the patient at risk of a delayed stroke [2]. Blood pressure is allow to remain elevated or may even be pharmacologically elevated during this period to promote blood flow through the cerebral vessels, helping to minimize the effects of vasospasm. Often patients are not awake enough to eat food or breathe on their own, thus requiring a ventilator to assist them in breathing and a feeding tube to administer nutrition [3]. As the patient improves, these mechanisms are often removed. The patient will remain in the Intensive Care Unit from admission until sometime after surgery, usually 3 weeks. Discharge often entails a rehabilitative facility depending on the neurological injury sustained.

Brain Tumors

Surgery offers the greatest chance for cure for many types of benign brain tumors, while it often serves as the crucial first step in tackling malignant tumors such as glioblastoma [4]. Depending on the size and location of the tumor, it may result in swelling of the brain, pressure upon other structures within the brain and/or increased intracranial pressure. Any of the above conditions often warrants surgery. Steroids, and prophylactic anti-epileptics are often required medications for treatment in conjunction with surgery. Radiation oncology is also very involved in the radiation planning procedure which is often employed adjunctively after surgery. After your surgery, the patient is admitted to the Intensive Care Unit, with close monitoring of vital signs and neurological status. Head of the bed elevation is encouraged to diminish post-operative swelling. Stitches or staples will have been used to close the incision and will be removed after 10–14 days. Pain medication will be given for incisional pain, steroids will be prescribed to diminish swelling, stool softeners will be given daily to prevent constipation and anti-seizure medications may also be needed. Discharge is usually either home or a rehabilitative facility after as soon as 2–3 days or as long as a week or two, depending on the neurological insult and amount of general deconditioning encountered.

Spine Surgery

Over one million spinal surgeries are performed each year in the United States [5]. Broadly, spine surgery can be performed for degenerative disease (spinal arthritis/herniated discs), spine tumors or scoliosis. If degenerative disease or a spine tumor causes an acute neurological deficit such as acute leg weakness or loss of bowel or bladder function, an emergency MRI will be obtained and emergent neurosurgical intervention may be indicated to decompress the spinal cord. Otherwise, spinal procedures are typically performed electively to ameliorate chronic symptoms such as leg pain as a result of degenerative disease, back pain or neurological symptoms from a spinal tumor, or to treat scoliosis. After any spinal procedure, the post-operative period is generally focused on carefully monitoring the neurological examination and tending to pain control [5]. The latter is often managed with narcotic pain medication and muscle relaxants. Physical therapy is also a crucial adjunct in recovering after spine surgery. Patients are often discharged after 2–3 days; rehabilitation may be indicated if a neurological deficit is sustained.

Traumatic Brain Injury (TBI)

The most common causes of TBI are closed head injury (fall / motor vehicle accident), open head injury (i.e. bullet wounds), and diffuse axonal injury (i.e. rapid back and forth movement of the brain within the skull) [6]. In all cases, the goal of management is to preserve blood flow to the brain and minimize the area of injury. Treatment may involve observation, placement of an external ventricular drain or bolt and/or surgery. Typically, if bleeding occurs inside in the brain itself, patients are observed. If their neurological examination is compromised, an external ventricular drain or bolt may be placed and medical measures to optimize the patient's elecrolytes during observation in an ICU setting are undertaken. Rarely, if a lot of swelling occurs around the blood in the brain, the patient may be taken to the operating room to remove a portion of the skull to allow the brain to safely swell. If bleeding occurs inside the skull but outside the brain itself (epidural or subdural), surgery is often performed to remove the blood clot. After surgery the patient will be admitted to the Intensive Care Unit, closely monitoring vital signs and neurological exam. Treatment for early signs of neurological compromise maximize a patient's chance for meaningful recovery. Intensive physical therapy and subsequent placement in a rehabilitation are often crucial to improve recovery if a sustained neurological deficit exists.

With all of the above conditions, some of the more common problems encountered after surgery include pain, infection, blood clots, lung infections, drug reactions, general infection, bleeding, slow recovery of bowels after surgery and problems with other organs, such as kidneys or heart.

Conclusion

The spectrum of neurological conditions and emergencies is extremely diverse. Appropriate assessment and neurological consultation is essential to good patient outcomes as many of these conditions depend on the rapid initiation of proper therapy.

References

1. Beresford L. Know your neurology. 2008. http://www.the-hositalist.org/details/article/188657/Know-Your-Neurology.html. Accessed 25 July 2013.
2. Kopitnik T, Samson D. Management of subarachnoid haemorrhage. J Neurol Neurosurg Psychiatry. 1993;56:947–59.
3. Goldberg C. Neurosurgical emergencies. Power point presented at the 4th annual symposium for the Mithoefer Center for Rural Surgery. 2009. Cooperstown, 17–18 May 2009.
4. American Cancer Society. Understanding cancer surgery: a guide for patients and families. American Cancer Society. 2011. Accessed 12 Aug 2013.
5. Katz J. Lumbar disc disorders and low-back pain: socioeconomic factors and consequences. J Bone Joint Surg. 2006;88 Suppl 2: 21–4.
6. Traumatic Brain Injury.com. http://www.traumaticbraininjury.com. 2004. Accessed 15 Aug 2013.

Chapter 7
Basic Neurosurgical Procedures

Rahul Kapoor, Caitlin Hoffman, Ibrahim Hussain, and Philip Stieg

Burr Hole

A burr hole is a small opening in the skull that is drilled to reach the dura mater, which is the outermost and thickest membrane enclosing the brain (Fig. 7.1). Several common indications that require a burr hole include elevated intracranial pressure (ICP) from infection, most commonly meningitis, trauma, and hemorrhage. A burr hole is also used to place intracranial pressure monitors, external ventricular drains, and brain oxygen monitors [3].

Procedure

Burr holes are most commonly placed at the bedside in the intensive care unit. After the patient is properly intubated for general anesthesia, sedated, and the head placed in a neutral position, a point 10 cm posterior to the nasion, which represents the intersection of the frontal bone and the two nasal bones, and 3 cm lateral to the midline, usually at the mid-pupillary line,

R. Kapoor, BS • C. Hoffman, MD • I. Hussain, MD
P. Stieg, PhD, MD (✉)
Department of Neurological Surgery, Weill Cornell Medical College, New York, NY 10065, USA
e-mail: pes2008@med.cornell.edu

A. Agrawal, G. Britz (eds.), *Comprehensive Guide to Neurosurgical Conditions*, DOI 10.1007/978-3-319-06566-3_7,
© Springer International Publishing Switzerland 2015

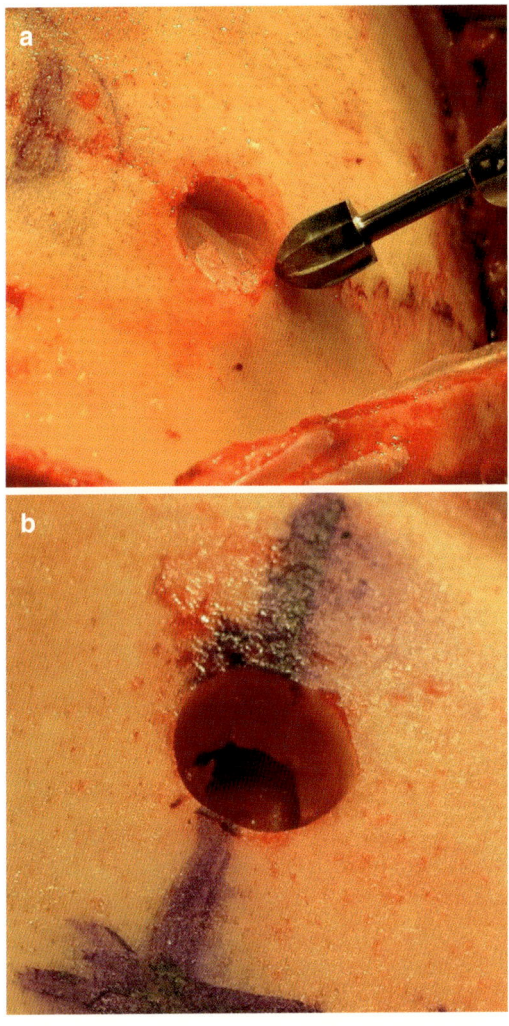

FIGURE 7.1 Burr hole. (**a**) Power drill being used to make burr hole. (**b**) Completed burr hole with dura mater at the base

is marked (Fig. 7.2). This is known as Kocker's point. A 2 cm area centered on this point is shaved, prepped and draped in sterile fashion. A linear incision is made in the scalp down to the

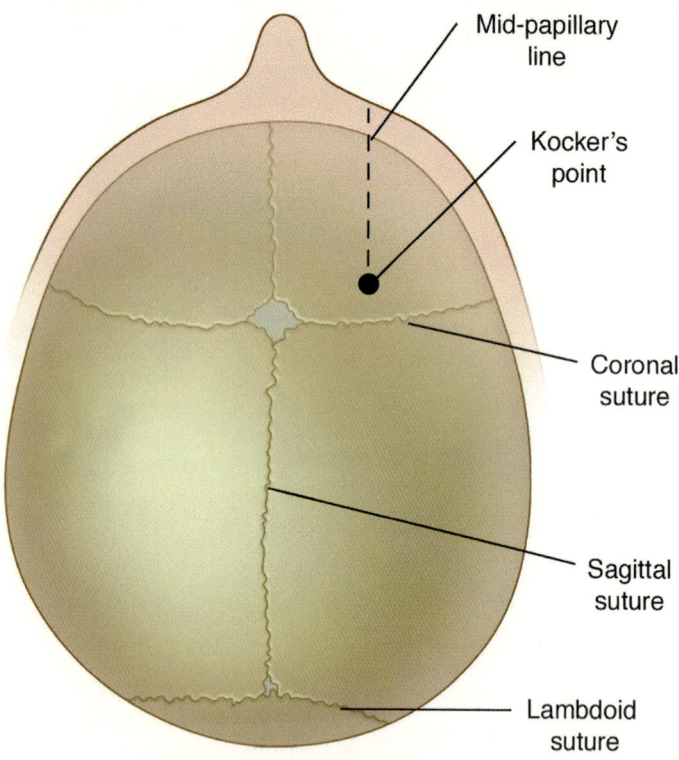

Mid-papillary
line

Kocker's
point

Coronal
suture

Sagittal
suture

Lambdoid
suture

FIGURE 7.2 View of the skull from the top with bony landmarks

skull. A hand-held twist drill is used to place a hole through the skull. The dura is opened sharply with a scalpel. For intracranial pressure, a ventricular catheter is then passed perpendicular to the skull down and aiming towards the ipsilateral medial canthus and mastoid process towards the ventricular space, which is a fluid filled space within the brain parenchyma, to a depth of 6.5 cm from the outer table of the skull (Fig. 7.3). The drain is used to measure intracranial pressure and to drain cerebrospinal fluid (CSF) to control pressure as needed. The catheter is then tunneled under the scalp, brought out from another puncture site, secured with multiple stitches, and sterilely connected to a drainage system [2–4] (Fig. 7.4).

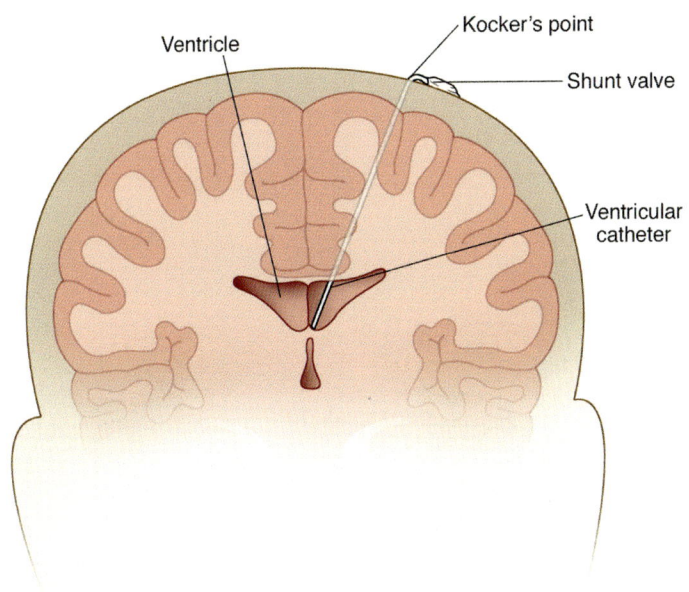

FIGURE 7.3 Ventricular catheter placed through the Kocker's point

Craniotomy

A craniotomy is a surgical procedure that requires removal of a bone flap to access the brain. Several common indications that require a craniotomy include removal of brain tumors, evacuation of intracranial hemorrhages, epidural and subdural hematomas, treatment of central pain syndromes (trigeminal neuralgia, hemifacial spasm), clipping of aneurysms, and removal of vascular malformations (arteriovenous

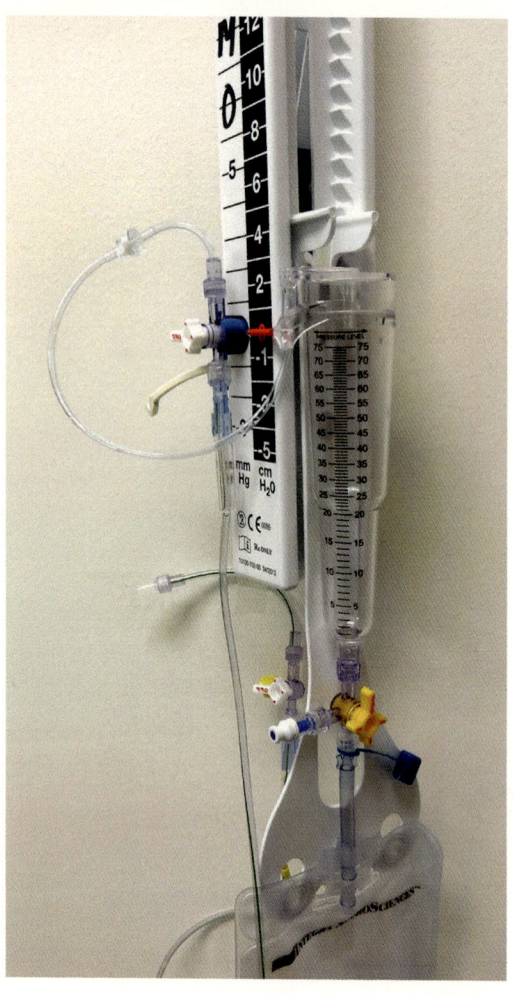

FIGURE 7.4 Sterile drainage system which connects to the ventricular catheter

malformations). Bone flaps can be removed from various parts of the skull and are dictated by the location of the pathology within the brain and skull. The names given to craniotomies include bifrontal, frontal, pterional, temporal, parietal, occipital, suboccipital, and far lateral, based on the location [3, 5].

Procedure

The patient is intubated and sedated under general anesthesia. A head clamp, commonly a frame with three points of fixation, is used to position the patient's head in a rigid position. The patient is positioned appropriately for the craniotomy which is dictated by the side and location of pathology. Often, computerized image guidance systems are used to specifically locate the lesion and plan the incision. Then, an incision is made in the scalp down to the bone, the pericranium is reflected, and a perforator drill is used to make burr holes in the skull. These holes are then connected with a specialized drill bit, and the bone flap is removed (Fig. 7.5). The dura is then incised sharply and reflected off the brain. The pathologic lesion is then removed, and the dura is closed over the brain primarily with suture material. If the dura cannot be closed primarily, grafts are sutured into the dura. The bone is then replaced with titanium plates in adults (Fig. 7.6) and sutures in young children. Finally, the scalp is closed over the bone [2–5].

Laminectomy

A laminectomy is a surgical procedure performed to remove part of the vertebral bone (commonly known as the backbone) called the lamina (Fig. 7.7). Several common indications that might require a laminectomy include spinal stenosis (which is a major cause for radiating leg pain and back pain), spinal disc herniation, tumor resection and decompression of the spinal cord [3].

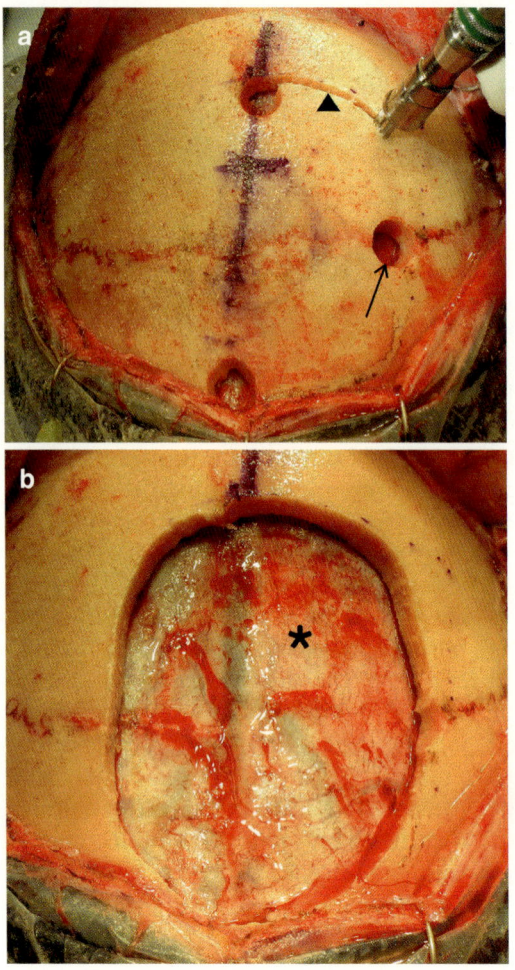

FIGURE 7.5 Craniotomy. (**a**) Burr holes connected by cuts in the skull (*arrow*) burr hole, (*triangle*) cut in skull. (**b**) Bone flap is removed exposing the dura mater which covers the brain (*star*) dura mater

Procedure

Precise surgical location is appropriated through the use of XRay. The patient is intubated, sedated under general anesthesia, and properly positioned. A midline incision parallel to

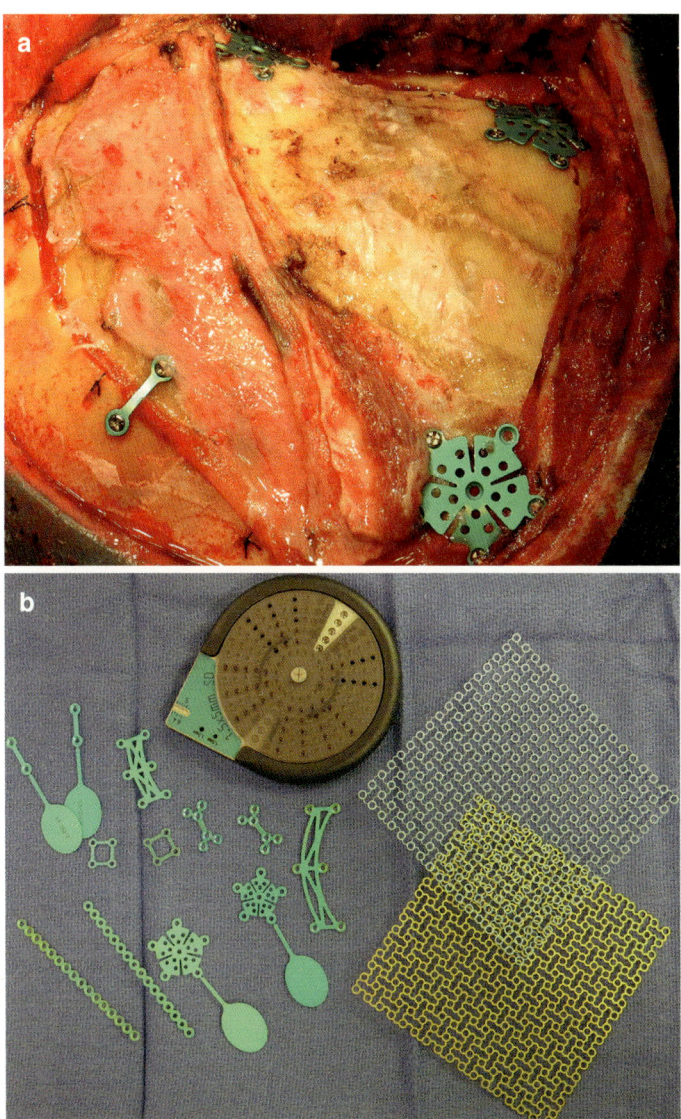

Figure 7.6 Craniotomy closure. (a) Bone secured after the surgery is completed using small titanium plates. (b) Titanium plates often used

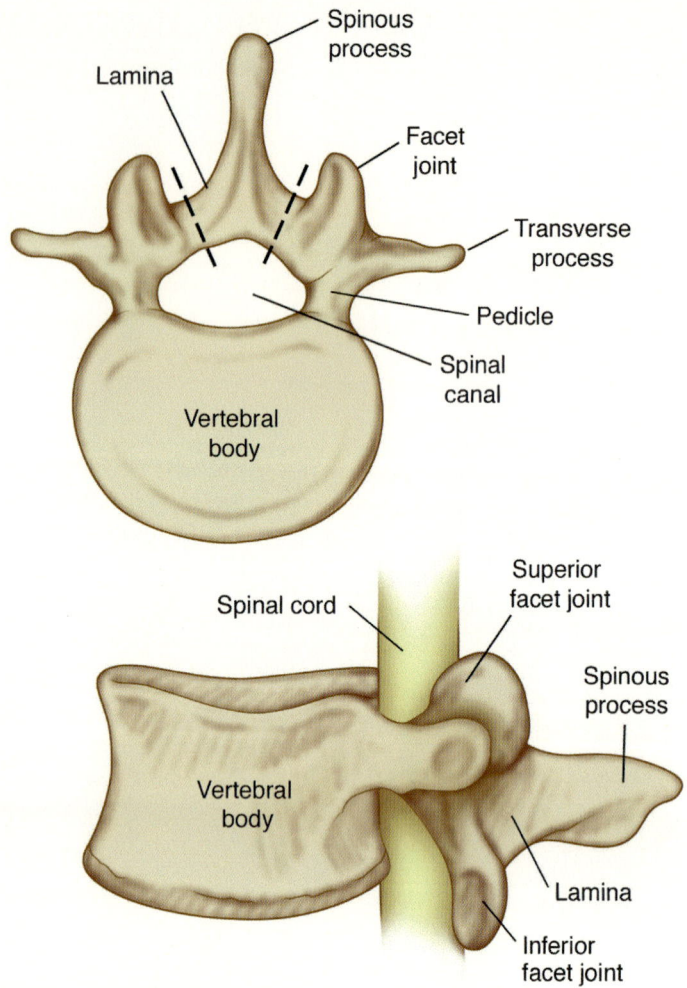

FIGURE 7.7 Typical vertebral body removal of the lamina and spinal process (laminectomy) provide access to the spinal cord. *Dashed lines* demonstrate the boundaries of the bone removal

the spinal column is made in the back, and the muscles are dissected down to the spinous process of the vertebra. The muscles are then dissected off of the lamina so that the lamina bone is exposed. A rongeur or drill is then used to remove the bone of the spinous process. A high speed drill is then used to remove the rest of the lamina bone to expose the underlying ligament. The ligament is removed and the dura encasing the spinal cord is exposed. Lamina bone is removed until the bilateral nerve roots are well decompressed as these are the common sites of compression and radicular nerve pain [3].

Shunt

A cerebral shunt is used to transport fluids, most commonly cerebrospinal fluid (CSF), from one location to another in order to decrease intracranial pressure (ICP). Several common indications that require a shunt include hydrocephalus, elevated ICP due to intraventricular hemorrhage, treated intracranial infection, or brain tumors causing CSF outflow obstruction [1, 3].

Procedure

After proper intubation, sedation, and positioning of the patient, a burr hole is drilled at the Kocker's point, 10 cm behind nasion and 3 cm lateral to midline. A shunt passer is then introduced under the skin from the point of the burr hole down to the abdomen. A second retroauricular incision may be needed and a removal guide passed to the abdomen. A final incision is made in the abdomen just lateral to the umbilicus. The abdominal muscles are dissected down to the inner fascial sheath, which is then incised and the peritoneum opened. A shunt catheter tube is then threaded through the shunt passers which are removed so the tubing is left in place below the skin. At the head, the dura is then opened and a ventricular catheter is passed through the brain into the ventricle, the fluid containing chambers within the brain. This catheter is then connected

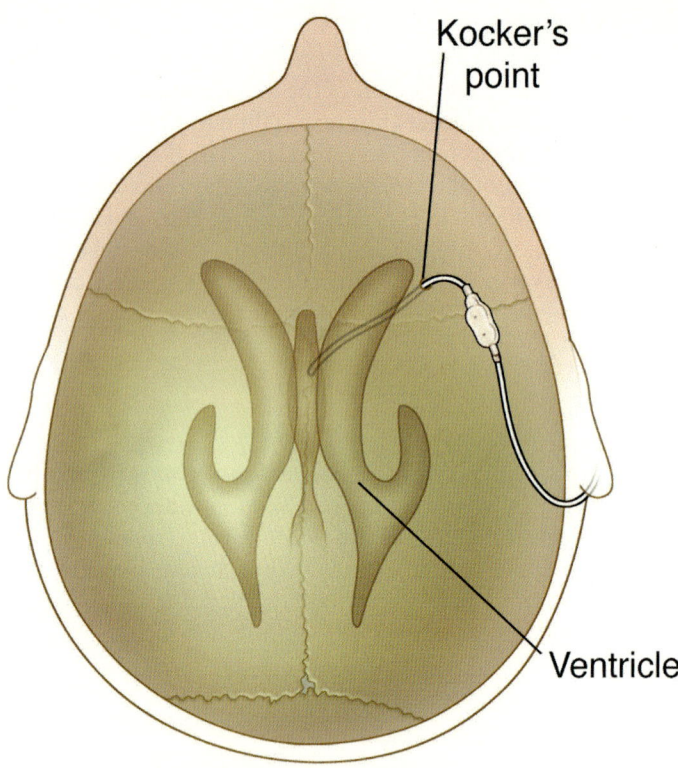

Kocker's
point

Ventricle

FIGURE 7.8 View of the skull and ventricles. Catheter is placed in the frontal horn of the ventricles and connected to the valve system. All tubing and valves are under the skin and are not visible to sustain sterility

to a valve. These valves are of varying pressures dependent upon the patient's intracranial pressure and the indication for the shunt. The distal end of the valve is connected to the peritonial end. Once CSF flow is established at the distal end of the tubing near the abdomen, the distal end of the catheter is then placed into the opening made in the peritoneum after the valve has been tunneled under the scalp (Figs. 7.8 and 7.9). All incisions are then closed [1, 3].

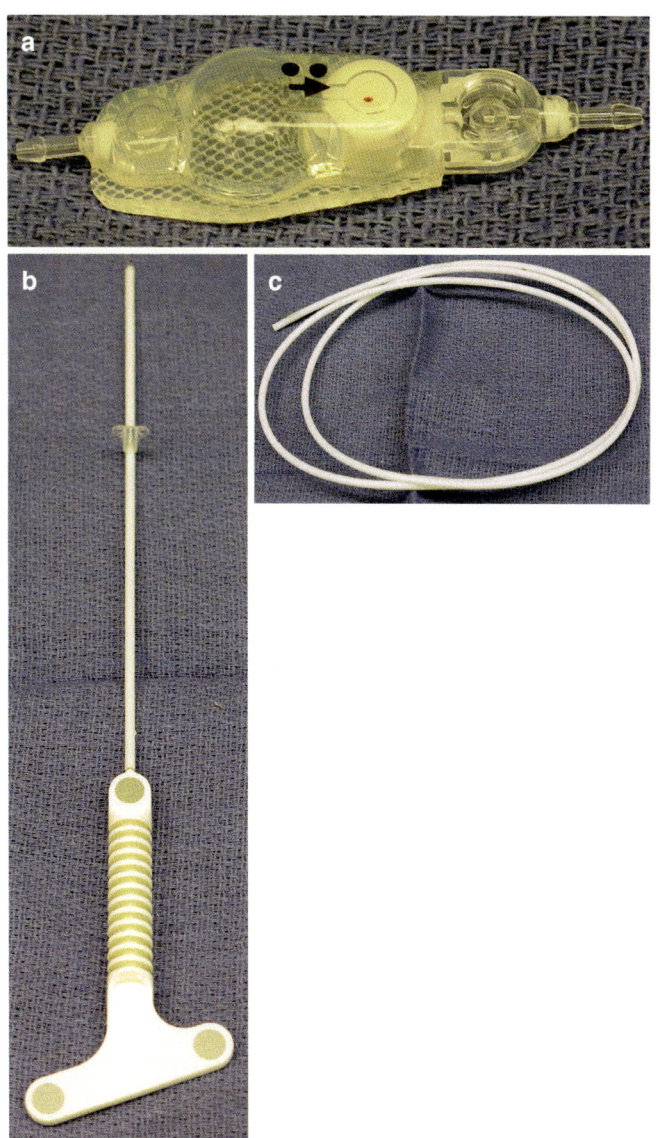

FIGURE 7.9 Shunt system. (**a**) Programmable shunt valve. (**b**) Ventricular catheter on a stereotactic stylet guidance system. (**c**) Distal end of the hunt tubing that runs under the skin and is placed in the abdominal cavity

References

1. Bergsneider M, Stiner E. Shunting. In: Winn HR, Berger MS, Dacey Jr RG, editors. Youmans neurological surgery. 6th ed. Philadelphia: Elsevier Saunders; 2011. p. 515–24.
2. Crowley RW, Dumont AS, McKisic MS, Jane Sr JA. Positioning for cranial surgery. In: Winn HR, Berger MS, Dacey Jr RG, editors. Youmans neurological surgery. 6th ed. Philadelphia: Elsevier Saunders; 2011. p. 442–6.
3. Greenberg MS. Handbook of Neurosurgery. 7th ed. New York: Thieme; 2010.
4. Rozet I, Vavilala MS. Risks and benefits of patient positioning during neurosurgical care. Anesthesiol Clin. 2007;25(3):631.
5. Warnick RE. Surgical complications of brain tumors and their avoidance. In: Winn HR, Berger MS, Dacey Jr RG, editors. Youmans neurological surgery. 6th ed. Philadelphia: Elsevier Saunders; 2011. p. 1285–92.

Chapter 8
Neurosurgical Emergencies

Neal Mehan and Raj K. Narayan

Depending on the disease, the treatment of brain and spinal cord problems can sometimes be very time-sensitive and require urgent treatment in order to preserve as much neurologic function as possible. Some of the commoner neurosurgical emergencies are from head and spinal cord injury, stroke and brain hemorrhages.

Traumatic Brain Injury

Traumatic brain injury is usually due to a fall, sports injury, assault or road traffic accident. In a battlefield setting it can also be due to blast injuries or gun and shrapnel wounds. Such injuries result in bleeding or bruising in the brain, or the formation of blood clots outside the brain that can cause compression of the brain. A head injury can result in a skull fracture. The fracture itself may not cause much damage unless it pushes the bone deeply into the brain. However, just the fact that the skull bone has been broken indicates that the impact

N. Mehan, MD • R.K. Narayan, MD (✉)
Department of Neurosurgery, Hofstra North Shore LIJ
School of Medicine, 300 Community Drive, 9 Tower,
Manhasset, NY 11030, USA
e-mail: rnarayan@nshs.edu

A. Agrawal, G. Britz (eds.), *Comprehensive Guide to
Neurosurgical Conditions*, DOI 10.1007/978-3-319-06566-3_8,
© Springer International Publishing Switzerland 2015

was severe. Just inside the skull one finds a fibrous membrane called the dura mater that is a sac that holds a watery fluid (cerebrospinal fluid). Skull fractures can be associated with bleeding in the space between the skull and the dura (epidural hematoma), between the dura and the brain (subdural hematoma) or inside the brain itself (intracerebral hematoma). In milder injuries, the brain may simply be bruised (contusion).

The goal in managing traumatic brain injury is to prevent further brain damage by maintaining a normal pressure level inside the skull (intracranial pressure). Because the skull can only contain a fixed amount of content, any increase in the size of the brain due to swelling, or due to a hematoma can result in increased intracranial pressure (ICP). This is normally below 20 mmHg. If the intracranial pressure becomes very elevated, the brain can be pushed downwards towards the opening in the bottom of the skull. This is called brain herniation and is life threatening. Emergency surgery may be needed to either remove a hematoma from the skull (craniotomy), or to remove the skull bone and allow the brain to expand till the swelling settles down (decompressive craniectomy). Signs of increased intracranial pressure include headache, nausea, vomiting, and decreased level of consciousness, which may progress into a coma. Basic treatments to decrease intracranial pressure include keeping the patient's head slightly elevated. Giving fluids with a high salt level (hypertonic saline) may also help to decrease swelling by reducing the water content in the brain (Fig. 8.1).

Spinal Injury

Spinal injury is one of the most devastating injuries seen in trauma patients. Spine injury occurs most commonly in sports injuries, motor vehicle accidents, and falls. The spine itself consists of multiple bones (vertebrae) that surround and protect the spinal cord. A pair of nerves exits at each level on each side. The results of spinal cord injury depends on the both the level and the severity of the injury. Below the level of injury the patient may have weakness or paralysis of the

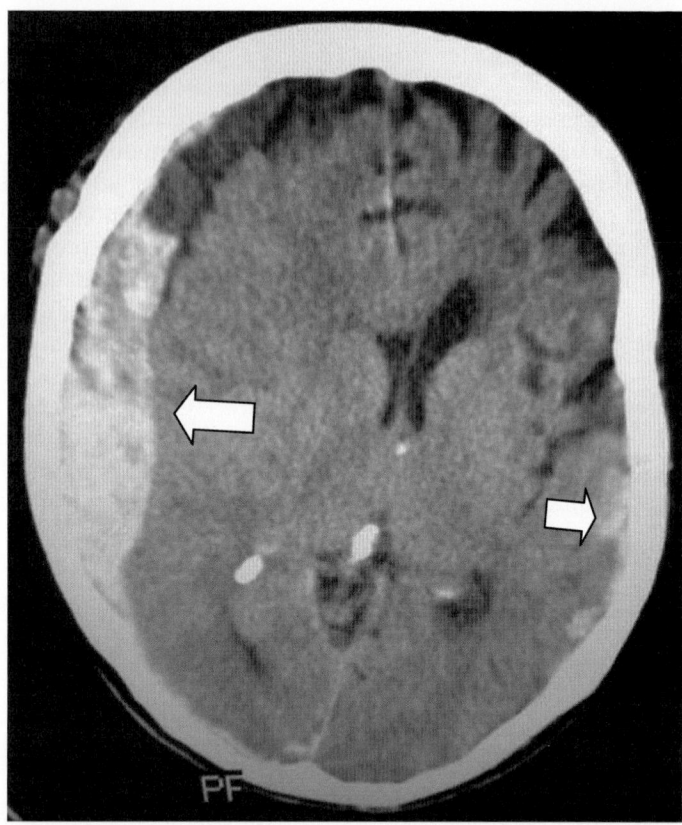

FIGURE 8.1 CT scan of the head in an elderly patient who fell. See the blood clot on the surface of the brain on the right side and some bruising of the brain (contusions) on the left. See also how the brain has been pushed from the right to the left (midline shift)

muscles, decreased sensation, and loss of bladder and bowel function. Therefore the higher the level, the more disabling the injury is likely to be. An injury in the neck or cervical spine would affect both the upper and lower extremities while one lower in the spine may only affect the lower extremities.

Fractures or a breakage of the spinal vertebrae can potentially result in spinal misalignment and instability. This misalignment can lead to compression of the spinal cord itself, or the exiting nerves and result in neurologic injury. Spinal cord injury can also occur from bruising or from compression of the cord by a hematoma. The primary goal in these situations is to restore the proper alignment of the spine and remove compression on the spinal cord and nerves. This can be done by pulling the spine straight (traction) or by surgery. The secondary goal after decompression is to restore the stability of the spine to prevent further spinal cord compression. In these cases, before definitive surgical stabilization can be undertaken, it is important to provide external stabilization of the spine with external braces to minimize motion to the area where the spine is unstable. These patients may have to be monitored in an intensive care unit to optimize blood pressure to ensure that the spinal cord is receiving enough blood to maximize the potential for recovery (Fig. 8.2).

Ischemic Stroke

An ischemic stroke occurs when the brain does not receive enough oxygen because of a lack of blood flow. The main cause of ischemic stroke is a blockage of a blood vessel from narrowing due to plaque formation, or a blood clot that forms at a plaque of a heart valve and flows downstream to occlude an artery that supplies the brain. Risk factors for developing strokes include advanced age, high blood pressure, high cholesterol, diabetes, blood clotting disorders, dehydration and smoking. The signs and symptoms of stroke will depend on what part of the brain is affected. Common symptoms include weakness on one side of the body, facial droop, and slurred speech. The onset is typically painless and the symptoms usually appear suddenly, although sometimes in a staggered manner. If a stroke is detected soon enough, a patient may qualify for a

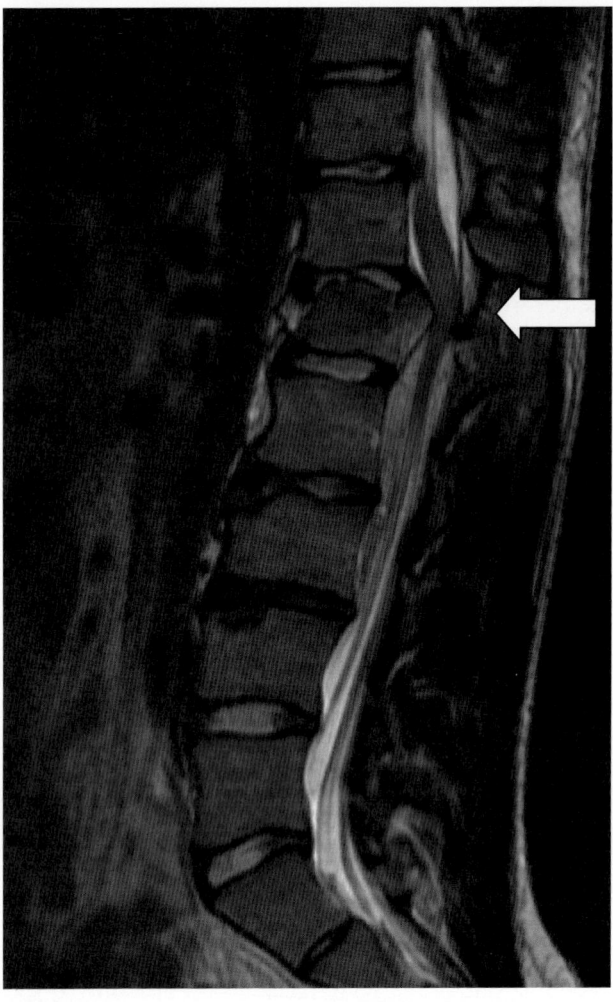

FIGURE 8.2 MRI of a patient who was involved in car accident. Note the displacement of the Lumbar 1 vertebra causing cord compression of the lower end of the spinal cord

drug (tPA) that can break up the blood clot and perhaps prevent brain injury. This medication has shown only to be beneficial if given within the first few hours of stroke onset and carries the risk of causing further bleeding into the brain. After a stroke, it is important to optimize blood pressure to maintain adequate blood flow in order to help with recovery.

Intracerebral Hemorrhage

Intracerebral hemorrhage or hematoma is bleeding within the brain tissue itself. It is a hemorrhagic stroke and is caused by rupture or leakage of smaller blood vessels in the brain. The symptoms caused by intracranial hemorrhage are dependent on the area of the brain that is affected and the severity of the neurological damage is often related to the size of the hemorrhage. Some of the common risk factors for developing intracranial hemorrhage are blood thinners, hypertension, diabetes, smoking, and excessive drinking. Treatment for intracranial hemorrhage is usually supportive. If the patient is on a blood thinner, this may have to be reversed with medications or special blood transfusions (fresh frozen plasma and platelets). In a few cases, surgery may be needed. The role of surgery in these cases is dependent on the location and severity of the hemorrhage. When the bleeding is deep within the brain, the risk of evacuation of the hemorrhage may outweigh the benefit of surgical removal because of injury to the normal brain tissue. If a hemorrhage is small enough, the brain will reabsorb the blood on its own over time. It is important in these cases to gradually control blood pressure to prevent further hemorrhage (Fig. 8.3).

Subarachnoid Hemorrhage

Sometimes, bleeding into the head can be from an aneurysm. These are blisters in the wall of the artery that can eventually burst releasing blood onto the surface of the brain. About a third of patients with subarachnoid hemorrhage will die immediately. Those who survive will need to be treated with

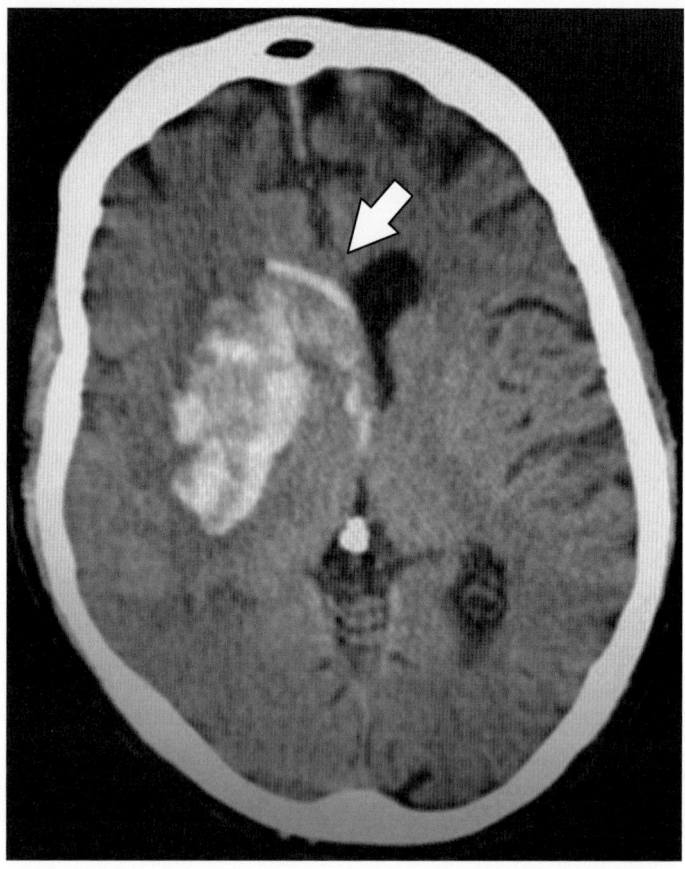

FIGURE 8.3 A CT of the head of a patient demonstrating a spontaneous intracerebral hemorrhage

surgical clipping or coiling of the aneurysm through a catheter in the groin. A less common problem is an arterio-venous malformation (AVM). This is a tangle of blood vessels that can also bleed like an aneurysm. These bleeds generally tend to be less severe than aneurismal bleeds. AVMs are treated with surgery or by focused radiation (radiosurgery) (Fig. 8.4).

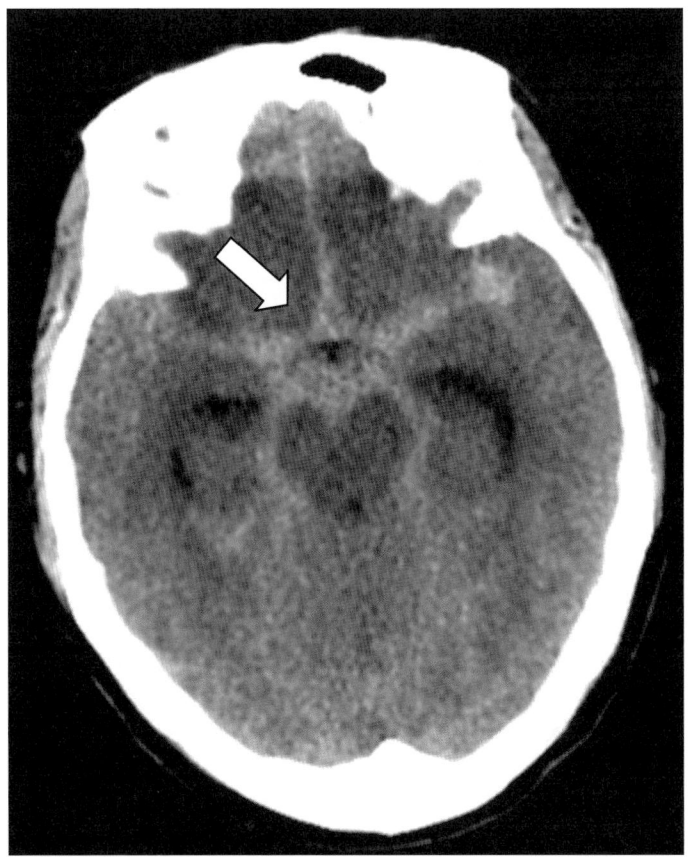

FIGURE 8.4 A CT of the head of a patient demonstrating subarachnoid hemorrhage

References

1. Saboe LA, et al. Spine trauma and associated injuries. J Trauma. 1991;31(1):43–8.
2. Hasler RM, et al. Epidemiology and predictors of cervical spine injury in adult major trauma patients: a multicenter cohort study. J Trauma Acute Care Surg. 2012;72(4):975–81.

3. Faul M, et al. Traumatic brain injury in the United States: emergency department visits, hospitalizations and deaths 2002–2006. Atlanta: Centers for Disease Control and Prevention, National Center for Injury Prevention and Control; 2010. p. 2–70.
4. Jauch EC, et al. Guidelines for the early management of patients with acute ischemic stroke a guideline for healthcare professionals from the American Heart Association/American Stroke Association. Stroke. 2013;44(3):870–947.
5. Sacco RL, et al. Risk factors. Stroke. 1997;28(7):1507–17.
6. Qureshi AI, et al. Spontaneous intracerebral hemorrhage. N Engl J Med. 2001;344(19):1450–60.
7. Narayan RK, Wilberger JE, Povlishock JT, editors. Neurotrauma. McGraw Hill

Chapter 9
Symptoms and Signs in Brain Disease

David B. Rosenfield

Symptoms Versus Signs

Patients can have multiple complaints. These complaints, referred to as "symptoms," are the main focus of the medical evaluation. This is why the most important issue when a patient is visiting the doctor may not be what a previous MRI or CAT scan or any particular test reveals but, rather, what actually bothers the patient. Then, after taking the patient's history, the physician determines whether the patient's symptoms do or do not relate to the findings on examination or testing.

Many times, patients have complaints that have nothing to do with their tests. For instance, a patient may have headaches and a cyst in their brain, but the two may not be related. Although no one should dismiss findings on any particular test, or on an examination (see below), the most important issue is what actually disturbs the patient, and then to be certain how, if at all, the patient's signs and testing relate to these complaints.

D.B. Rosenfield, MD
EMG and Motor Control Laboratory, Speech and Language Center, Neurological Institute, Houston Methodist Hospital, Weill Medical College of Cornell University, Houston, TX, USA
e-mail: drosenfield@houstonmethodist.org

A. Agrawal, G. Britz (eds.), *Comprehensive Guide to Neurosurgical Conditions*, DOI 10.1007/978-3-319-06566-3_9,
© Springer International Publishing Switzerland 2015

"Signs," as opposed to "symptoms," are the objective abnormalities the physician detects on examination. These can include: delineation of weakness, abnormal coordination, abnormal pupil size or response to light, eye movements and other abnormalities. Again, the major issue is to intercalate how the patient's complaints (i.e., symptoms) relate to the physician's detection of signs (i.e., objective abnormalities).

A good example is in order. If a tree falls on your roof, you may have broken shingles and a leak from the ceiling. However, the two may not be related—the leak may have nothing to do with the broken shingles but, rather, results from damage to the support system of the gutters or damage to the flashing around the chimney.

Put another way, abnormalities in structure (e.g., broken roof shingles) can be independent of abnormalities in function (e.g., ceiling leak). The same is true in brain disease: an abnormality in structure (e.g., seen on an MRI of the brain) may not relate to abnormality in function (e.g., weakness of the arm).

Symptoms in Brain Disease

One of patients' most common neurological complaints is headache. Headaches can be mild or severe, last seconds, minutes, hours or days, be in different locations on the head and often are quite frightening. Sometimes, these are associated with tingling sensations in the back or front of the head (tingling usually implies neck or facial nerve disorder), and other headaches can be associated with ocular or facial pain.

It is important to note the brain has no pain receptors. That is why Alzheimer's disease and Parkinson's disease do not hurt (nor does it hurt to think, a cerebral activity). This is also one reason why brain tumors can be so serious—one does not feel the tumor.

The only pain receptors within the cranial vault are in the covering of the brain (i.e., meninges, infection or irritation of which can cause meningitis) and the walls of arteries, which can swell in migraine or stretch from a tumor or hydrocephalus. Most headaches, such as muscle tension headaches, emanate from the neck region. Cervical compromise can cause headaches—this is one reason why there are head/neck rests on the seats of automobiles: to alleviate flexion/extension cervical compromise in an accident, and decrease risk of headaches and neck injury.

If someone has a headache that does not go away, or is significantly disturbed by this pain and, especially, if it is the worse headache the patient has previously experienced, one should rule out a cerebral cause of the pain, especially recognizing that bleeding (e.g., vascular abnormality, arteriovenous malformation, aneurysm) in the brain area, including an area referred to as "subarachnoid space," can irritate the covering of the brain (e.g., dura, meninges) and cause head pain. Also, tumors or cysts can obstruct spinal flow in the brain, or stretch arteries and these, too, can cause headache.

When people have headaches due to brain disease, or even due to neck disease, it is the additional taking of the history from the patient as well as the physical/neurological examination that assists the physician in determining whether the head pain reflects brain compromise or neck compromise, or something else, such as infected bone, eroding sinuses, etc.

Patients can also complain of difficulty thinking or abnormal language, which are always indicative of brain compromise. Problems with thinking, whatever the cause, always reflect some problem with the brain, since the brain is where thinking occurs. If someone has an abnormality of language (e.g., using incorrect words, putting words together in an abnormal grammatical context, or difficulties with language comprehension), this, too, signifies brain compromise, usually in what is referred to as the language-dominant hemisphere (i.e., right-handed people have language dominance in the left side of their brain; left-handed people have less language dominance in the left side of the brain and the stronger is their left-handedness, the greater the dominance shifts to the right side of the brain).

When people have intermittent difficulty with thinking or language, or with vision or weakness, one should suspect an intermittent problem with the "pump or the pipes" (e.g., respectively, abnormalities in cardiac function or blood flow to the brain) or seizures (see below). Alterations in smell sometimes signify brain compromise but more often signify damage in the sinuses or nasal passageways.

Complaints of areas of blindness, especially if this involves both eyes, raise strong suspicion of brain compromise. Double vision, although it can be a symptom of a "lazy eye" or neuromuscular disease causing weak eye muscles, should raise suspicion of brain disease.

When one has visual loss or blurriness, or double vision, it is important for the patient to cover one eye and then the other, to ascertain whether the symptom reflects brain or eye disease (i.e., if one has a visual defect from brain disease, that defect is usually present in each eye, regardless of whether one eye is manually covered; if one has double vision, and sometimes the patient is not certain regarding the accuracy of this complaint, the double vision should normalize if one eye or the other is covered).

As noted above, intermittent symptoms can reflect seizures which, in turn, can reflect brain tumor, stroke or various types of epilepsy. It is important to note not only what happens when the patient has a seizure, (i.e., whether they lose consciousness, fell, extended their limbs, shook their limbs, lost bowel or bladder control, tongue biting) but also what was the first symptom, if any, that heralded the onset (called the "aura") of the seizure, since this assists the physician in localizing the abnormality in the brain causing the seizure. For instance, auras of nausea or abdominal upset can reflect seizure foci in certain portions of the temporal lobe, shaking of the hand can reflect particular abnormalities in the motor strip in the frontal lobe, etc.

Another symptom important regarding seizures is whether the patient was confused following the seizure. When cardiac compromise causes patients to lose consciousness, these episodes are usually brief (i.e., cardiac syncope) and the patient is alert post-episode. However, seizures (especially generalized seizures involving both sides of the brain) often render people confused following the seizure. The presence or absence of confusion following loss of consciousness helps differentiate syncope from seizure.

Patients can complain of abnormal speech, with intact word choice and grammar, but their sounds are slurred. This can be a sign of brain compromise and signify brain location of disease. It is important when one has disturbance of language or speech or both, to mention to the physician whether your comprehension was good during this episode (e.g., can be abnormal in language disturbances but will be normal in pure speech disturbance) and whether people in your vicinity could recognize the words or whether the words made no sense (i.e., "Where is the falred?" instead of, "Where is the book?").

Patients can also complain of weakness or sensory abnormalities in their limbs, another possible signature of brain disease, especially if the patient complains of weakness in an arm and leg on the same side, often signifying cerebral disease on the contralateral side (spinal cord pathology may also have to be excluded).

Signs in Brain Disease

After completing the history, the neurologist/neurosurgeon performs a neurological examination. After obtaining the necessary vital signs (i.e., height, weight, blood pressure, pulse, respiratory rate), the physician evaluates several parameters, looking for objective neurological signs, trying to relate these to the patient's complaints.

It is important to know whether the patient is alert, oriented, and has normal language, speech and memory, all of which can be abnormal in brain disease, as noted above.

The physician assesses gait, an abnormality of which can reflect brain, spinal cord, nerve, or muscle compromise. If gait is abnormal in the setting of disturbance of thinking, one considers degenerative brain disease, obstruction to spinal fluid flow (e.g., hydrocephalus), tumor and other diseases.

The physician also looks for atrophy, tremor at rest, fasciculations (muscle twitches), rigidity and slowness of movement, which can be seen in multiple instances of brain disease.

The physician evaluates the patient for proprioception (i.e., recognition of position sensation) and pallesthesia (i.e., vibration sensation), abnormalities of which usually reflect nerve or spinal cord compromise, not brain disease.

Finger-to-nose and heel-to shin maneuvers should be performed fluidly and without tremor. Abnormalities can reflect disturbance in the cerebellum of the brain, be it degenerative disease, tumor or stroke.

Pupils should be round, equal and react well to light, whether the light is shined in the eye being directly examined or in the consensual eye (i.e., shine a light in the right eye, the left pupil should constrict). If the light reflex of the pupils is abnormal, especially if there is an abnormality on one side but not the other, compromise of brain and arterial supply to the brain should be considered. Brain disease should also be considered if one of the pupils is significantly different (i.e., greater than 2 mm) in size than the other, often raising suspicion of aneurysm.

Eye movements should be fluid and conjugate (i.e., move together) in all directions of gaze, whether to one side or the other, up or down. If there is dysconjugate movement (i.e., one eye does not move in cadence with the other) or if there are jerking movements to one side (i.e., "nystagmus"), this can reflect brainstem disease, especially if inner ear disease has been excluded.

As noted above, testing the visual fields is also important, abnormalities of which can reflect brain disease, be it from tumor or stroke.

Facial muscles and power and corneal reflexes (e.g., touching one of the corneas with a wisp of cotton should produce blinking in both eyes) should be bilaterally symmetrical.

Biceps, triceps, brachioradialis, knee and ankle reflexes, as well as jaw jerk reflexes, all elicited with a reflex hammer briskly tapping the implied tendons, should be symmetrical and not too brisk. When they are very brisk, especially if they continue to "jerk" after the reflex is elicited (known as "clonus"), they can signify brain (or spinal cord, except for the fact that spinal cord compromise does not affect the jaw jerk reflex) compromise. When these reflexes are brisk, it is especially important to note whether there is a Babinski response, meaning the big toe extends when a noxious stimuli scratches the bottom of the foot.

Power should be carefully assessed. It is not necessary to examine every muscle, but is important to assess the basic set of proximal (i.e., upper muscles of arm and leg), distal (i.e., lower muscles of arm and leg) and muscles that flex and extend the limbs. Then, the pattern of weakness is merged with the findings on reflex assessment to decide whether there is an abnormality in the brain, spinal cord, nerve or muscle realm.

Putting It All Together

All diseases are either congenital or acquired, a perspective usually readily obtainable from the patient's history. If the disease is acquired, whether that disease reflects brain compromise or disturbance of other organs, the disease usually reflects trauma, infection, vascular compromise, degenerative disturbance, tumor or abnormalities in the toxic/metabolic realm. The above delineation of symptoms and signs, while not considered total in scope, provides a good filter for the physician to achieve a working diagnosis (or diagnoses), which, depending upon the nature of the complaint(s), can warrant particular diagnostic tests further to elucidate the cause of the patient's symptoms and thus assist with focused treatment.

Suggested Reading

1. Rowland LP, Pedley TA. Merritt's neurology. 12th ed. Philadelphia: Walters Kluwer, Lippincott, Williams & Wilkins; 2010.

Chapter 10
Sports Related Concussion Injuries

Kenneth Podell

Introduction

Sports-related concussion (SRC) is one of the biggest health concerns today for youth athletes. Just a few short years ago an athlete would have returned to a game after sustaining a concussion even if symptomatic and applauded for their courage. The times have changed and SRC are finally recognized for being a legitimate brain injury requiring proper diagnosis and treatment.

Definition

A concussion is a form of mild traumatic brain injury caused by external trauma to the brain and results in a metabolic disruption of brain functioning. Signs and symptom onset is typically rapid but can evolve over several hours that spontaneously remit over time.

K. Podell, Ph.D.
Houston Methodist Concussion Center,
6560 Fannin Street, Ste 1840, Houston, TX 77030, USA
e-mail: kpodell@houstonmethodist.org

A. Agrawal, G. Britz (eds.), *Comprehensive Guide to Neurosurgical Conditions*, DOI 10.1007/978-3-319-06566-3_10,
© Springer International Publishing Switzerland 2015

Mechanism

A direct blow to the head can cause a concussion, but direct force to the face or even the body is enough to illicit a concussion. There are three mechanisms that result in a concussion: (1) acceleration/deceleration (the brain rocking back and forth and striking the skull); (2) translational energy (when two objects hit the energy "pulses" through the brain distorting its shape); and (3) Rotation of the brain places strain on the center parts of the brain (much like a twisted knee).

Epidemiology

The actual rate of SRC is unknown because many go unreported. However, an estimated 1.6–3.8 traumatic brain injuries (all levels) occur annually in the USA [9, 13]. It is estimated that over 400,000 SRCs occur annually in 7.5 million student-athletes in the USA [4, 11, 20].

The rate of SRC varies by gender, sport and level of participation with "contact" sports having the highest rate. SRC is most common in American style football where upwards of 40 % of HS football players will sustain a concussion. However, the rate of concussions is comparatively higher in females who play the same or similar sports as men [7, 15]. Concussion frequency is 6–25 times more likely in competition than in practice depending upon age, gender and sport [12, 15].

Signs and Symptoms

SRC are characterized by a set of signs and symptoms that differ between individuals (see Table 10.1). Headache, sensitivity to light or sound, dizziness with poor balance and mental fogginess are some of the more common symptoms acutely, with headache, memory and concentration problems,

TABLE 10.1 Concussion-related symptoms

Headache	Vomiting	Dizziness
Nausea	Balance problem	Fatigue
Trouble falling asleep	Irritability	Feeling mentally "foggy"
Sleeping more/less than usual	Sadness	Difficulty concentrating
	Nervousness	Difficulty remembering
Sensitivity to light	Feeling more emotional	Visual problems
Sensitivity to noise	Numbness/tingling feeling slowed down	
Drowsiness		

sleep problems and fogginess more common later in the concussion.

Loss of consciousness (LOC) rarely occurs following a SRC (only 10 %), and when it does, is often very brief (<1 min). Also, LOC is a poor predictor of severity or prognosis for recovery from a SRC. Rather, impaired memory around the event, severity of headache and number of other symptoms are better at predicting recovery from SRC [5, 19].

Gender is a factor in the severity of SRC symptoms [1, 2, 10] and cognitive deficits [3]. Women, as a group, often have more symptoms and more severe cognitive deficits (memory and concentration) that take longer to recover from than do males.

Immediate Care

Individuals suspected of having a concussion should be evaluated by a health care provider (HCP) experienced in concussion management. Often a school athletic trainer is the first to evaluate an athlete. Determining if a serious neck/

TABLE 10.2 Signs and symptoms indicating a more serious brain injury may be present

1. Increased sleepiness or confusion (cannot be fully aroused from sleep)

2. Worsening headache

3. Continued vomiting

4. Stumbling and incoordination

5. Sudden numbness or weakness in the arms or legs

6. Unintelligible speech or dramatic personality change

7. Unequal pupil size

8. Very stiff neck with limited range of motion

9. Seizure/Convulsions or "fits"

spine injury was sustained is done first. Next, the HCP will determine if a concussion was sustained using a symptom questionnaire, balance assessment, and short mental tests that can easily be administered at the scene. The player should be monitored after a diagnosed concussion for any worsening or development of symptoms that indicate a more serious brain injury (a bleed). Table 10.2 is a common list of symptoms and signs to look for in cases of a more serious brain injury. Typically, brain imaging such as a CT scan is not required, but the decision will be made by a treating doctor. However, when in doubt, always seek medical care.

Recovery

SRC is a transient disorder from which 90 % will recover from fully within 30 days. Age, gender, and certain medical history determine the length of time it takes to recover. Concussions are highly individualistic and predicting recovery time is difficult. Often, younger athletes take longer to recover [22]. It can take two weeks for a concussion to resolve, but sometimes it can take upwards of over 1 month. However, such factors as gender, number of prior concussions, history of ADHD, LD, or psychiatric illness or increase the recovery period from SRC.

About 10 % take longer than 1 month and even a smaller percentage have a longer period of SRC symptoms and cognitive problems referred to as a post-concussive syndrome (PCS). There appear to be several factors that contribute to PCS such as concussion severity, number of prior concussions, history of ADHD, LD or psychiatric disease and psychological factors [8, 17].

Treating a Concussion

After any neurological emergency has been ruled out rest is the best medicine for treating an acute concussion. Contrary to a popular wives-tail, it is alright to allow a child with a concussion to sleep at night without waking him/her up every hour as long as he/she has been cleared by a HCP. Long stretches of sleep at night with a few shorter naps in the day (not in the early evening) is often the quickest way to help the brain heal. Often times it is better to allow the child to stay home from school and rest for a few days immediately after the concussion because the loud and bright school environments often worsen concussion symptoms. Besides, the student often has trouble focusing, paying attention and remembering in classes in the early stages of a concussion. In addition, we often recommend that the student not be responsible for homework or quizzes and tests for a period of time after the concussion because of concentration and memory problems with worsening headaches. A gradual increase in classes and homework is often the best way to return a child to school following a concussion (see Table 10.3).

Over the counter pain medication can be used after a concussion to help with headache pain. No aspirin for the first 48 h because of its blood thinning properties. Some doctors will not use NSAIDs for the first 48 hours (e.g., ibuprofen or naproxen sodium) for the same reason. Thus, acetaminophen is the OTC pain medication of choice. Some physicians will

TABLE 10.3 Sample of a gradual return to school program for concussed student-athletes

Step 1: emphasize cognitive and physical rest	No physical activity
	Rest body and brain as much as possible
	May need to stay home from school
Step 2: open for modified daily class schedule	No participation in PE or physical activity
	Reduced work load and/or no quizzes or exams
	Extra time on exams and assignments if given
Step 3: possible return to full day of school	May engage in light physical activity after being cleared by a health care provider
	Gradually increase amount of assignments and examinations
	Extra time on assignments and exams
Step 4: reduction of accommodations and return to moderate physical activity	May engage in moderate physical activity
	May take tests
	Should be allowed extra time on exams
Step 5: full academic load	May engage in physical activity without any restrictions
	May return to school full time without any restrictions

use a variety of prescription medications to treat headache pain, however, there are no set guidelines.

Return to Play Guidelines

Athletes who sustain a concussion should not be allowed to return to contact sports until they are symptom free, cognitively intact (or return to baseline), have intact balance, and are functionally normally at school. The typical guideline suggestions a period of gradually increasing cardio-aerobic

TABLE 10.4 Example of a typical return to play exercise program for sports concussion

Step 1
Light aerobic activity for 15 min keeping your heart rate between 50 and 60 % of TMHR* (e.g., walking, stationary bike, elliptical machine, treadmill, jogging and hand bike) for ____ days. No weight lifting at this step.
Step 2
Moderate physical activity for 20 min keeping your heart rate between 65 and 70 % of TMHR (e.g., running, light weights, push-ups & sit-ups) for ___ days. No weight lifting at this step.
Step 3
Moderate physical activity 25–30 min keeping your heart 80 % of TMHR (e.g., running, light weights, push-ups & sit-ups) for 1 day.
Step 4
Intense physical activity for at least 30–35 min keeping your heart rate between 80 and 85 % of TMHR (e.g., non-contact practice with sport specific drills).
Step 5
1 day of full practice (with contact).
Step 6
Return to competition.

*Theoretical maximal heart rate

activity, followed by sport specific drills, weight lifting, non-contact practice, contact practice and finally competition (see Table 10.4 for an example). The athlete must maintain a symptom free status through each step. If not, the athlete rests until symptom free and starts again.

Long-Term Effects

There has not been enough time to adequately research the long-term effects of concussions. However, there is mounting evidence that a history of multiple concussions effects memory and speed of thinking decades later in life [6]. Some research has shown changes in brain functioning after a season of heading in soccer or football [14, 16]. But no study has shown changes in school grades.

Protective Equipment

There is no such thing as a concussion proof helmet as long as there is an opportunity for the brain to move inside of the skull. Research shows difference in linear force reduction between different current helmets in the lab but not in reported concussions in football [18, 21]. Mouthpieces are great for protecting the oral cavity and jaw but do nothing to reduce concussions. Soccer helmets are not effective in reducing concussions, but likely reduce lacerations or contusions to the scalp and skull.

State Laws

Presently, all 50 states have statues regulating sports concussion. While there is a lot of variability, most laws have rules about education, evaluating concussions on the sideline or before returning to play, not allowing players to return in the same competition, and guidelines for return to play. The following is an interactive map for all of the state laws passed: http://www. edweek.org/ew/section/infographics/37concussion_map.html.

Preventing Concussions

There are some precautions one can take to help reduce the chance of having a concussion:

1. Ensure that the helmet fits snuggly and is in good condition (outside and inside padding). The helmet should not move independently of the head.

TABLE 10.5 Websites with important educational materials about concussions

1. Center for Disease Control and Prevention: http://www.cdc.gov/concussion/

2. Sports Legacy Institute: http://www.sportslegacy.org/

3. Think First: http://concussioneducation.ca/

4. Concussionwise: http://www.concussionwise.com/

5. The American Academy of Neurology: http://www.aan.com/Concussion

2. Neck strengthening can reduce the amount of movement of the brain and force that travels into the brain. It also reduces the effects of whiplash and neck injuries.
3. Educate the student-athlete, parent, coaches and medical professionals. This will help everyone know what a concussion is, what to do when someone experiences one, how to evaluate and how to return safely and make informed decisions about return to play.
4. Do not return to play prematurely.

Several websites offer educational videos, information, and downloadable materials about concussions for various interested parties (Table 10.5).

References

1. Bazarian JJ, Blyth B, Mookerjee S, He H, McDermott MP. Sex Differences in Outcome after Mild Traumatic Brain Injury. J Neurotruama. 2010;27:527–39.
2. Berz K, Divine J, Foss KB, Heyl R, Ford KR, Myer GD. Sex-specific differences in the severity of symptoms and recovery rate following sports-related concussion in young athletes. Phys Sportsmed. 2013;41(2):58–63.
3. Broshek DK, Kaushik T, Freeman JR, Erlanger D, Webbe F, Barth JT. Sex differences in outcome following sports-related concussion. J Neurosurg. 2005;102(5):856–63.

4. Centers for Disease Control and Prevention. Nonfatal traumatic brain injuries from sports and recreation activities: United States, 2001–2005. MMWR Morb Mortal Wkly Rep. 2007;56(29):733–7.

5. Collins MW, Inverson GL, Lovell MR, McKeag DB, Norwig J, Maroon J. On-field predictors of neuropsychological and symptom deficit following sports-related concussion. Clin J Sport Med. 2003;13(4):222–9.

6. DeBeaumont L, Brisson B, Lassonde M, Jolicoeur P. Long-term electrophysiological changes in athletes with a history of multiple concussions. Brain Inj. 2007;21(6):631–44.

7. Dick RW. Is there a gender difference in concussion incidence and outcomes? Br J Sports Med. 2009;43 Suppl 1:i46–50.

8. Eisenberg MA, Andrea J, Meehan W, Manix R. Time interval between concussions and symptom duration. Pediatrics. 2013;132(1):8–17.

9. Faul M, et al. Brain injury in the United States: emergency department visits, hospitalizations and deaths 2002–2006. Atlanta: Centers for Disease Control and Prevention, National Center for Injury Prevention and Control; 2010.

10. Frommer LJ, Gurka KK, Cross KM, Ingersoll CD, Comstock RD, Saliba SA. Sex differences in concussion symptoms of high school athletes. J Athl Train. 2011;46(1):76–84.

11. Gessel LM, Fields SK, Collins CL, Dick RW, Comstock RD. Concussions among United States high school and collegiate athletes. J Athl Train. 2007;42(4):495–503.

12. Kontos AP, Elbin RJ, Fazio-Sumrock VC, Burkhart S, Swindell H, Maroon J, Collins MW. Incidence of sports-related concussion among youth football players aged 8–12 years. J Pediatr. 2013;163(3):717–20.

13. Langlois JA, Rutland-Brown W, Wald MM. The epidemiology and impact of traumatic brain injury: a brief overview. J Head Trauma Rehabil. 2006;21:375–8.

14. Lipton ML, Kim N, Zimmerman ME, Kim M, Stewart WF, Branch CA, Lipton RB. Soccer heading is associated with white matter microstructural and cognitive abnormalities. Radiology. 2013;268(3):850–7.

15. Marar M, McIlvain NM, Fields SK, Constock RD. Epidemiology of concussions among United States high school athletes in 20 sports. Am J Sports Med. 2012;40:747–55.

16. McAllister TW, Flashman LA, Maerlender A, Greenwald RM, Beckwith JG, Tosteson TD, et al. Cognitive effects of one season

of head impacts in a cohort of collegiate contact sport athletes. Neurology. 2012;78:1777–84.

17. McCrea M, Guskiewicz K, Randolph C, Barr WB, Hammeke TA, Marshall SW, et al. Incidence, clinical course, and predictors of prolonged recovery time following sport-related concussion in high school and college athletes. J Int Neuropsychol Soc. 2013;19:22–33.

18. McGuine TA, Hetzel S, McCrea M, Brooks MA. Characteristics associated with the incidence of sport-related concussion in High School Football Players: A multifactorial prospective study. Am J Sports Med. 2014;42:2470–8.

19. Meehan WP, Mannix RC, Stracciolini A, et al. Symptom severity predicts prolonged recovery after sport-related concussion, but age and amnesia do not. J Pediatr. 2013;163(3):721–5.

20. Patel DR, Shivdasani V, Baker RJ. Management of sport-related concussion in young athletes. Sports Med. 2005;35(8):671–84.

21. Rowson S, Daniel RW, Duma SM. Biomechanical performance of leather and modern football helmets. J Neurosurg. 2013;119:805–9.

22. Zuckerman SL, Lee YM, Odom MJ, Solomon GS, Forbes JA, Sills AK. Recovery from sports-related concussion: days to return to neurocognitive baseline in adolescents versus young adults. Surg Neurol Int. 2012;3:130–4.

Chapter 11
Radiotherapy for Brain and Spine Disease

John P. Kirkpatrick and Fang-Fang Yin

Introduction

Radiation therapy is a key element in the integrated management of primary and metastatic tumors of the central nervous system [1]. This chapter discusses the application of radiotherapy, alone and in combination with surgery and chemotherapy, in the treatment of metastases to the brain (the most common malignant brain lesion), primary malignant gliomas (the most common malignant primary brain tumor) and metastases to the osseous spine.

J.P. Kirkpatrick, MD, PhD (✉)
Department of Radiation Oncology, Duke University
Medical Center, 3085, Durham, NC 27710, USA

Department of Surgery, Duke University Medical Center,
Durham, NC, USA

Duke Cancer Institute, Duke University Medical Center,
Durham, NC, USA
e-mail: john.kirkpatrick@dm.duke.edu

F.-F. Yin, PhD
Department of Radiation Oncology, Duke University
Medical Center, 3085, Durham, NC 27710, USA

Duke Cancer Institute, Duke University Medical Center,
Durham, NC, USA

A. Agrawal, G. Britz (eds.), *Comprehensive Guide to Neurosurgical Conditions*, DOI 10.1007/978-3-319-06566-3_11,
© Springer International Publishing Switzerland 2015

Brain Tumors

Radiotherapy Techniques

In the modern practice of radiation therapy, ionizing radiation, typically in the form of high-energy x-rays, is accurately and precisely delivered to treat tumors or benign lesions while sparing surrounding normal tissues [2]. Radiation kills tumor cells by damaging DNA though the generation of free radicals, not by heating tissue [3]. In the United States, most radiation therapy uses high-energy x-rays produced by linear accelerators, though radioactive isotopes and protons are also utilized.

While a variety of equipment and techniques are used to deliver therapeutic radiation, all systems share some common features. Effectively planning a radiation treatment requires that the patient be held in a fixed position (immobilization) that can be reproduced faithfully during radiation treatment. After immobilization, x-ray, CT and/or MR images are taken to identify the target for radiation and determine its precise location in space (localization.) These planning images are often combined with diagnostic images (for example, PET or MR images) and the target and normal structures drawn by the radiation oncologist to generate a 3D model of the patient and tumor. Then, radiation fields are designed to cover the tumor while excluding normal tissues. Typically, multiple intersecting beams are employed to deliver a high dose at their intersection while spreading out the radiation in normal tissues, with extremely accurate calculation of the actual dose delivered. The choice of the specific radiation technique and doses is driven by the need to deliver an adequate dose to the target while keeping the dose to normal tissues within recognized limits [4]. Treatment may be delivered either in a single or multiple doses, depending on the size and location of the lesion, the disease type and the objective of treatment. In all cases, the patient is precisely positioned in the desired position on every day of radiation therapy and the position confirmed. Needless to say, this is a complex and demanding process, relying on robust quality assurance procedures and a multi-disciplinary team composed of physicians, physicists, dosimetrists, radiation therapists and nurses.

Specific examples of brain radiotherapy techniques follow below:

Whole-Brain Radiotherapy (WBRT)

Radiation therapy to the entire brain uses a relatively simple technique, typically employing two parallel opposed lateral fields with the patient supine. In preparation for planning and treatment, the patient is positioned on a head rest or immobilized using a custom-molded thermoplastic mask or simply tape (Fig. 11.1a). Prior to treatment, X-ray or CT images are acquired and a treatment plan is developed using opposed megavoltage x-ray beams (Fig. 11.1b). The central axis of the beam is typically placed near the eye to minimize the divergence of radiation beams into the lenses. In addition, the face and anterior eyes/lenses are blocked and the beam "shaped" using lead blocks or a multi-leaf collimator. At the time of treatment, the position of the treatment field is verified by imaging the treatment fields with the patient appropriately positioned on the radiation treatment table.

3D and Intensity-Modulated Radiation Therapy

In 3D treatment of brain tumors, the lesion is drawn on multiple CT or MRI slices to create a three-dimensional structure. This structure may be expanded several millimeters to centimeters in each direction to yield a target volume. The treatment planner then sets up multiple beams in the computer, each of which is sized, shaped and weighted to achieve the desired dose to the target while minimizing dose to the normal brain. During treatment, lead blocks or thin metal leaves in the linear accelerator are used to achieve the desired shape of the radiation beams. In intensity-modulated

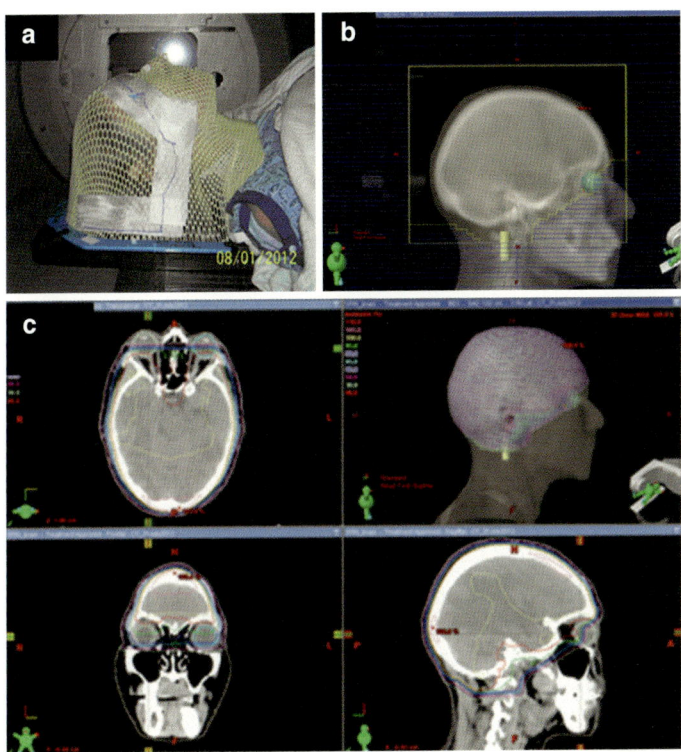

FIGURE 11.1 Typical patient immobilization and field set-up for whole-brain radiotherapy (WBRT) via opposed lateral fields. (**a**) Custom headholder with field shape outlined on mask, (**b**) multileaf collimator outline (*dark blue lines*) and (**c**) radiation dose distribution – starting from upper right-hand corner and moving clockwise: 3D rendering of dose distribution for sagittal, coronal and axial cross-sections (Reprinted from Kirkpatrick et al. [5]. With Permission from Elsevier)

radiotherapy (IMRT), the shape of the beam is continuously adjusted by adjusting these metal leaves, permitting the dose to be precisely varied within the target volume. This "dose painting" is particularly useful when treating irregularly shaped targets that wrap around critical normal structures, such as the brain stem or optic nerves.

Intracranial Stereotactic Radiosurgery (SRS)

In SRS of brain lesions, a high dose of radiation is delivered in a single fraction or a few fractions with rapid dose fall-off from the periphery of the target lesion into the surrounding normal brain. While a variety of radiotherapy systems, e.g., GammaKnife (Elekta), CyberKnife (AccuRay), Novalis Tx (Varian Medical Systems and BrainLab), are utilized in intracranial SRS, all share some common features [6]. SRS systems exhibit high accuracy (<1 mm deviation) for patient positioning and dose delivery. Typically, a patient is immobilized in a removable, semi-rigid plastic head mask (Fig. 11.2a) or a head ring fixed to the patient's skull. The target for radiation is precisely identified using fine-cut CT scans fused with MR images and occasionally functional imaging modalities, such as PET.

In a collimator-based linear-accelerator system, such as the Novalis Tx, a typical treatment plan for an ellipsoid lesion, such as a small brain metastasis, consists of three to five noncoplanar conformal arcs (as illustrated in Fig. 11.2b) yielding the conformal dose distribution shown in Fig. 11.2c. Multiple intensity-modulated beams are often used for treating irregularly shaped targets and/or those that are immediately next to critical organs, such as the brainstem. The correlation between the patient geometry (and/or immobilization device geometry) and the treatment machine geometry is achieved through two different approaches: (1) matching the geometry of the immobilization device with the machine isocenter through dedicated measurement devices with the assistance of room lasers; (2) matching planning/simulation images with treatment images acquired using an imaging device mounted in the treatment room (or machine) while the patient is on the treatment table. Both approaches are able to achieve localization accuracy of about 1 mm. Radiation delivery consists of multiple beams intersecting at a single point (isocenter), shaped by fixed diameter cones and delivered in multiple arcs, dynamically conformal arcs continuously shaped by a multi-leaf collimator or multiple intensity-modulated beams. In the CyberKnife system, multiple collimated small-diameter beams are delivered to an intracranial lesion using a linear accelerator attached to a highly mobile robotic arm.

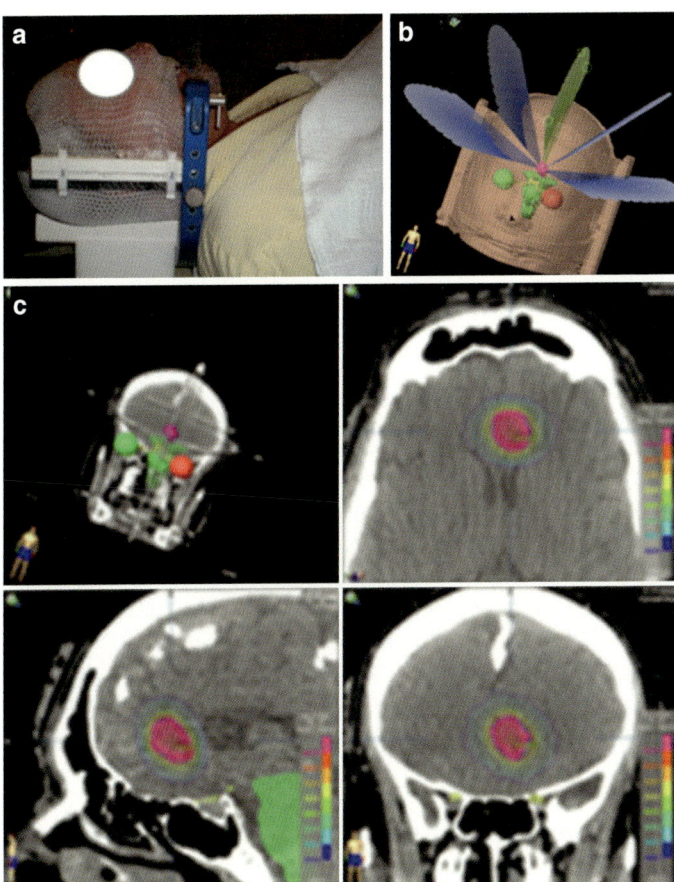

FIGURE 11.2 Example of patient immobilization and field set-up for stereotactic radiosurgery (SRS) via dynamic conformal arcs to a left frontal lobe metastasis. (**a**) Custom U-frame mask, (**b**) multiple arc paths and (**c**) radiation dose distribution – starting from upper left-hand corner and moving clockwise: 3D rendering of dose distribution for axial, coronal and sagittal cross-sections (Reprinted from Kirkpatrick et al. [5]. With Permission from Elsevier)

In contrast, the GammaKnife system uses hundreds of gamma-ray sources (Co-60) precisely intersecting at a single isocenter. This yields a small spherical or ellipsoid high-dose cloud whose diameter is determined by the size of the collimator opening. Dose fall-off from the cloud into the surrounding tissue is extremely rapid. Treatment of irregular and/or large targets is achieved by "packing" together multiple dose "clouds," positioned in the target by precisely repositioning the patient over the course of a treatment session.

Brain Metastases

Primary cancer metastatic to the brain (brain metastases) is the most common malignant lesion in the brain, developing in over 200,000 cancer patients in the United States each year [7]. While brain metastases from lung, breast, kidney and skin (melanoma) are most frequently encountered, virtually any histology from any anatomic suite can metastasize to the brain. The optimal management of brain metastases is controversial, given the improved control of extracranial disease and increased longevity after cancer is diagnosed, multiple tumor and patient factors influencing prognosis, and the many treatment options. Treatment typically consists or whole-brain radiotherapy, radiosurgery, surgical resection or some combination of these modalities, as described below. Chemotherapy does not yet play a significant role in the management of brain metastases [8].

WBRT with and Without Surgery

Whole-brain radiotherapy is widely employed for the treatment of patients with brain metastases. WBRT can temporarily halt the growth of brain metastases, gradually reducing mass effect and neurologic deficits and extending life. However, there is a substantial risk of recurrence and neurologic death, and WBRT is typically delivered with palliative intent. Acute side effects of WBRT include complete hair loss and mild scalp erythema and pruritus in nearly all patients, occasional sensation of fullness in the ears and parotid swelling, and mild anorexia and moderate fatigue which can be severe in the debilitated and/or elderly patient [9]. Steroids (primarily dexamethasone) should be given judiciously, using the lowest dose to control symptoms while carefully managing the many potential side effects. Prophylactic anti-epileptic drugs should not be routinely administered [10].

The long-term impact of WBRT on neurocognition and quality-of-life is a common concern of patients and their families. A frequently cited study of patients from Memorial Sloan-Kettering with single brain metastases treated with WBRT reported that "radiation-induced dementia" was observed in 5/47 patients at 1-year (11 % crude rate.) Note that four of the five patients who developed dementia were treated with a high dose per fraction (three 5- to 6-Gy fractions) and that the other received a concurrent radiosensitizer. In contrast, none of the 15 patients treated in ten 300 cGy fractions developed dementia. Today, patients with brain metastases treated with brain metastases typically receive ten 300 cGy, fourteen to fifteen 250 cGy or twenty 200 cGy fractions, though shorter or longer courses can be utilized. While data from low-grade primary tumors suggest that a more protracted course affords better preservation of neurocognition [11, 12], the optimal dose/fractionation regimen for brain metastases has not been established [13].

Studies of single brain metastases treated with WBRT with and without surgery have yielded conflicting results [14–16]. For example, a randomized trial of WBRT alone versus surgery plus WBRT suggests that surgery be considered in all surgical candidates with a single resectable lesion [16]. The rate of recurrence at the original site of metastasis was significantly lower in patients who were resected and irradiated (20 versus 52 %), overall survival was much higher and functional independence longer compared to those who received

WBRT alone. In contrast, another randomized study of WBRT with and without surgery in 84 patients with single brain metastases showed no significant difference with the addition of surgery.

Surgery with and Without WBRT

The resection of a brain metastasis can reduce the pressure on adjacent structures, recurrence of disease at the resection cavity and in other areas of the brain occurs frequently. In a trial of patients with a solitary brain metastasis randomized to surgery with or without WBRT, recurrence of tumor anywhere in the brain was far less frequent in the group receiving WBRT (18 % versus 70 % [17]). The addition of WBRT reduced the risk of recurrence at both the original site of the metastasis and at other sites in the brain, and these patients were less likely to die of neurologic causes. However, the study showed no significant difference in overall survival with or without WBRT. A subsequent study from the European Organization for Research and Treatment of Cancer (EORTC) randomized over 300 patients with one to three brain metastases to observation versus WBRT after either surgery or SRS [18]. The primary endpoint was deterioration in performance status. Recurrence at the resection site and the uninvolved areas of the brain was significantly higher when WBRT was omitted, and patients receiving WBRT were less likely to die of intracranial disease. However, the study found no difference in time to deterioration of performance status or in overall survival.

WBRT with and without SRS

The Radiation Therapy Oncology Group randomized 333 adult patients with one to three brain metastases treated with WBRT to SRS within 1 week of completing WBRT versus observation (RTOG 9508 [19].) Local control was significantly improved in the group undergoing SRS (82 versus 71 % at 1 year), though recurrent disease anywhere in the brain was not significantly better. Nonetheless, median overall survival was significantly higher with the addition of SRS in patients with a single brain metastasis patients <65 years old with controlled extracranial disease and Karnofsky performance status ≥70, and patients with brain metastasis ≥2 cm in greatest diameter. In addition, patients receiving treated with SRS exhibited significantly reduced steroid use and less deterioration in Karnofsky performance status than those who did not. Rates of acute and late toxicities were quite similar between the two groups, though SRS carried an approximate 0.5 % monthly rate of radionecrosis.

SRS with or without WBRT

SRS alone with close follow-up to detect and treat recurrent disease has been suggested as an alternative to whole-brain radiotherapy, as it potentially avoids neurocognitive and systemic side effects encountered with treatment of the entire brain. On the other hand, omitting WBRT carries a significantly higher risk of recurrence, which in turn may result in increased neurocognitive deficits. Sneed et al. [20] performed a retrospective analysis of 569 patients from ten institutions treated with SRS alone versus SRS with up-front WBRT. There was no significant difference in the median overall survival time for patients receiving SRS alone versus SRS and WBRT.

In a study from Japan [21], patients with one to three brain metastases were randomized to receive SRS alone versus SRS and WBRT. The addition of WBRT significantly improved both control at the site of the original metastases (89 versus 73 % at 1 year) and at distant sites in the brain (58 versus 36 % at 1 year.) However, overall survival was not different with SRS alone versus SRS and WBRT. As measured by mini-mental status exam (MSE), neurocognition did not differ between these arms [22], though MMSE is admittedly not a sensitive instrument for detecting changes in cognition.

In contrast a study from M. D. Anderson [23] randomized 58 patients with brain metastases to receive SRS alone versus SRS and WBRT, focusing on neurocognitive decline as measured by a comprehensive battery of tests. Four months after SRS, neurocognitive decline was substantially higher in the group receiving WBRT – 52 versus 24 %. Similar to other studies, the 1-year freedom from recurrence anywhere in the brain was 27 % for SRS alone versus 73 % for SRS plus WBRT. However, median overall survival was substantially poorer than expected in patients treated with WBRT. As the neurocognitive decline was measured at a time when many of the patients in the WBRT group were close to death, the results of this study are somewhat difficult to interpret.

SRS with Surgery

Following resection of a single brain metastasis, the surgical cavity alone can be treated with radiosurgery, omitting whole-brain radiotherapy, with the objective of decreasing the high rates of local recurrence observed with surgery alone [17] and avoiding the side effects of WBRT [24]. For example, Choi et al. irradiated 120 resection cavities in 112 patients with brain metastases [25]. At 1 year, the rate of recurrence at the cavity was 9.5 % while the rate of distant failure in the brain was 54 %. They also examined the effect of irradiating only the resection cavity versus the resection cavity expanded by 2 mm and found that the rate of local failure at 1 year was significantly lower in the 2 mm and that no significant difference in toxicity was observed as a function of resection margin.

Decision-Making

All patients with brain metastases should be treated with some form of radiation therapy. In determining which patients should be treated with surgery before or after radiation, there are generally six features to consider, as follows: comorbidities, patient prognosis, size, location and number of metastasis, and patient goals for treatment. In general, patients with a poor prognosis due to fulminant disease outside the brain or other comorbidities should be treated with radiation only, as the time to recover from surgery is generally a minimum of 3–6 weeks and surgery imparts risks that may increase the recovery time. Given increasing tumor burden and decreasing maximum tolerated dose for radiosurgery as tumor diameter increases, many patients with tumors >3 cm and most patients with lesions >4 cm diameter should be considered for surgery. It is also generally accepted that patients with a single metastasis or more than one metastasis that can all be accessed through a reasonable sized craniotomy should be considered for surgical resection. Finally, patient's preference should always be a factor in the decision given the lack of Level I data to support specific recommendations, particularly with regard to the choice between surgery plus radiation versus radiation alone. This discussion will involve the neurosurgeon, radiation oncologist, the patient and other members of the care team.

Primary Brain Tumors

Malignant Gliomas

Anaplastic astrocytomas and glioblastomas (WHO Grade III and IV malignant gliomas, respectively) account for about two-thirds of primary malignant brain tumors in adults with an annual incidence in the U. S. of approximately six cases/100,000 person-years [26]. While meningiomas are more frequent, these are typically benign tumors [26] and the discussion in this section will focus on the management of the far more aggressive malignant gliomas. Malignant gliomas arise from neuroepithelial tissue and with a peak incidence in the sixth decade of life. The cause of most cases of malignant gliomas is unknown in more than 90 % of cases, though exposure to ionizing radiation and certain genetic syndromes are associated with an increased risk of this disease [27].

Surgery

Maximum safe resection of malignant glioma is a key element in the management of malignant gliomas, as outcomes appear to be more favorable in patients undergoing a gross or near total resection compared to minimal debulking or biopsy alone [28]. However, there are no randomized control studies proving the superiority of a gross total resection and it is unlikely that such a trial would be performed. With surgery alone, median progression-free and overall survival are on the order of only a few months, as tumor cells are present well beyond the gross lesion. Thus, surgery and radiotherapy are typically both utilized, as described below.

Radiotherapy

Radiation therapy following surgical resection of malignant gliomas has been a recommended component of the management strategy since the 1970's, as the combination of surgery and RT improved overall survival over surgery alone [29, 30]. Subsequent studies suggested that a total dose of around 60 Gy, typically administered at 2 Gy per day, improved survival compared to lower total doses [31, 32]. Trials to improve outcome by dose escalation using conventionally fractionated RT [33], hyperfractionation [34], brachytherapy [29, 35] or a stereotactic radiosurgery [36] boost have not revealed a benefit to increasing dose beyond 60 Gy. Thus, standard RT typically consists of thirty 2.0 or thirty-three 1.8 Gy daily fractions to a total dose of 59.4–60 Gy delivered over a 6–7-week period. However, there is evidence in elderly patients, that treatment at a slightly higher dose per day for a significantly shorter period (e.g., 40 Gy delivered over 3 weeks) may yield a reasonable outcome [37].

Though the entire brain was initially irradiated due to the concern about the invasion of tumor cells throughout the brain, various trials showed no significant differences in outcome when the volume of brain irradiated was reduced [38, 39]. In addition, most failures occur within 2–3 cm of the enhancing lesion on CT or MRI scans and a distant failure is usually associated with a local recurrence [38, 40]. Thus, in order to avoid toxicity associated with whole-brain irradiation to 60 Gy, the current practice is to irradiate only the involved part of the brain. Typically, the initial target for irradiation is the volume of brain exhibiting T2 hyperintensity on MRI expanded by approximately 2 cm, followed by a "boost" of an additional 14–14.4 Gy to the contrast-enhancing residual lesion and/or resection cavity on T1-weighted MRI imaging. In order to minimize the volume of normal brain irradiated and to keep the dose to critical structures within tolerance, multiple shaped, intersecting radiation beams are employed and intensity-modulated radiotherapy is often utilized.

Surgery, Radiotherapy and Chemotherapy

Meta-analyses of the outcome in patients with malignant glioma treated with or without nitrosureas suggested a small, but significant, benefit from the addition of these intravenous agents [41, 42]. However, an EORTC trial in which patients with glioblastoma were randomized to receive RT (60 Gy in 2 Gy daily fractions) with or without temozolomide (TMZ), demonstrated that the addition of TMZ yielded significantly improved overall survival [43]. Patients expressing lower levels of the enzyme responsible for repair of DNA damage, MGMT, exhibited a much more favorable response, though an improvement in survival was noted in the RT/TMZ arm even in those patients with unfavorable MGMT status. Likewise, while younger age, performance status and increased extent if resection were associated with better outcome, the addition of TMZ conveyed improved survival in all prognostic groups. Consequently, the standard of care for adult patients with newly diagnosed glioblastomas includes maximum safe resection followed by conventionally fractionated radiotherapy with concurrent and adjuvant chemotherapy.

Even with the "optimum" combination of surgery, radiotherapy and chemotherapy, the virtually all patients with malignant glioma recur [43]. A variety of novel approaches are under trial to improve outcome in newly diagnosed glioblastoma, and enrollment in these trials is essential to identify more effective treatment. Given the extremely high rates of recurrence in malignant gliomas, improved treatment of recurrent disease is also a matter of great interest. Bevacizumab has been approved by the FDA for treatment of recurrent disease based on the results of phase II trials [44–46] and SRS, alone [47] or, particularly, in combination with bevacizumab [48–50], may offer benefits in this setting. Randomized trials testing the efficacy of SRS and bevacizumab (RTOG 1205) are underway.

Spine and Spinal Cord Tumors

Radiotherapy Techniques

External-Beam Radiotherapy (EBRT)

EBRT for spine tumors are typically utilizes one of three techniques: (1) a single radiation beam entering posteriorly (PA field, Fig. 11.3a), (2) two opposed radiation beams entering anteriorly and posteriorly (AP-PA fields) or (3) three or more radiation beams, often shaped by multi-leaf collimators (conformal 3D beams, Fig. 11.3b) All of these EBRT techniques result in irradiation of entire vertebral body, with the spinal canal/cord receiving the full dose of radiation. If control of the tumor is the primary objective of treatment, multiple modest doses of radiation are used (typically, ranging from five 4 Gy daily fractions up to twenty 2 Gy fractions.) Alternatively, if pain relief is the goal, it may be possible to treat with a single 8 Gy fraction, though this may limit durability of response. Both the PA and AP-PA fields are relatively quick to design and deliver. The PA field may reduce dose to the chest and abdomen, but is limited in the depth of treatment, particularly for lesions located in the lumbar spine. AP-PA fields are capable of treating deep lesions but deliver

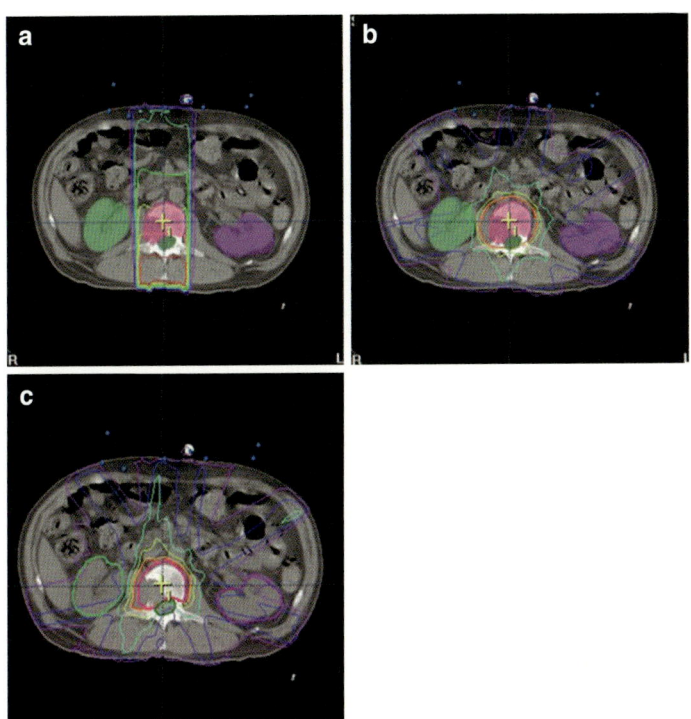

Figure 11.3 Typical axial radiation dose distributions for (**a**) external-beam radiotherapy to the spine via posterior-anterior fields and (**b**) multiple 3D conformal beams, (**c**) spinal stereotactic radiosurgery via intensity-modulated radiotherapy (Reprinted from Kirkpatrick et al. [5]. With Permission from Elsevier)

higher radiation doses to the viscera. In contrast, 3D conformal EBRT plans are more complex to plan and execute but significantly reduce the maximum dose to adjacent organs (see Fig. 11.3b)

Spinal Radiosurgery

For metastatic disease involving one or a few contiguous vertebral bodies, SRS can be utilized to treat the osseous spine while sparing the spinal cord with one or a few high dose fractions. To do so, it is essential to employ intensity-modulated radiation therapy (IMRT) or volumetric modulated arc therapy (VMAT) to treat the concave target while minimizing dose to the canal [51–54], as shown in Fig. 11.3c. As in intracranial radiosurgery, key elements of spinal SRS include high-resolution imaging for planning, immobilization and imaging for position verification and adjustment immediately before and during treatment [55, 56].

Primary Spine Tumors

Primary tumors of the spinal cord, nerves and meninges are rare, comprising less than 5 % of primary CNS tumors. In adults, the most common primary tumors are meningiomas, nerve sheath neoplasms and ependymomas [26]. These tumors are often associated with severe symptoms, including pain, parathesias, paralysis and loss of bowel/bladder continence, with the severity of signs and symptoms related to the extent of tumor and the specific site of cord affected. Tumors of the spinal canal and cord may be surgically resected to relieve mass effect and reduce the severity of symptoms, to obtain a tissue diagnosis and/or, in the case of benign tumors such as spinal myxopapillary ependymomas, to achieve a cure. Following surgery, radiation therapy is frequently recommended in the setting of residual and/or malignant disease, typically covering the entire circumference of the spine and canal at the involved levels. Irradiation of the entire craniospinal axis is appropriate in rare circumstances and carries significant morbidity. Alternatively, radiotherapy may be the sole treatment modality in patients who are not surgical candidates because of the extent of systemic disease, short life expectancy, potential morbidity and/or refusal of surgery. Again, the radiation field typically includes the entire level of the involved cord/canal plus a margin of one vertebral body above and below this level. SRS is typically reserved for spinal nerve schwannomas with minimal intra-canlicular extension.

Metastatic Disease to the Osseous Spine

While primary tumors of the boney spine are rare, metastases to the spine are quite common, with about 10 % of all cancer patients developing symptomatic spinal metastases and a far greater number have occult disease [57–59]. The most frequent presenting symptom of osseous spinal metastases is back pain [59–61], though paralysis, parathesias, radicular pain and bowel/bladder incontinence are seen in many cases, particularly when the spinal canal is compromised and the cord compressed. Radiographically, lytic lesions and pathologic fracture are readily apparent on plain films and CT scans, though MR imaging is most sensitive for identifying more subtle lesions and defining the extent of cord/canal compromise and epidural disease. Time is of the essence in diagnosing and treating malignant spinal cord compression, necessitating the emergent initiation of steroids, concurrent consultation with radiation oncologist and spinal surgeon, and rapid intervention [58, 62–64].

In *appropriate* patients with neurologic compromise from metastatic disease to the boney spine, surgical decompression followed by radiation therapy is the treatment of choice, as shown in a randomized trial [65] of patients with malignant spinal cord compression treated by surgical decompression followed by RT versus RT alone. The surgical arm exhibited significantly superior outcome, including ambulation rate following treatment (84 versus 57 %), duration of ability ambulate (median 122 versus 13 days), return of ambulation after treatment in non-ambulatory patients (62 versus 19 %), and urinary continence (74 versus 57 %,). However, the selection criteria for this study were quite restrictive, excluding patients with radiosensitive tumors, short life expectancy and multifocal disease, limiting the eligible patient population to only 10–15 % of the patients with malignant spinal cord compression [66]. A retrospective matched pair analysis of patients with malignant spinal cord compression (without these strict exclusion criteria) treated with decompressive surgery and RT versus RT alone showed no significant difference in any functional outcome [66].

Patients who are not candidates for surgery may be appropriately treated with radiotherapy alone, assuming that a diagnosis of malignancy has been established. However, patients frequently present with a symptomatic spinal lesion as the first manifestation of malignant disease and then issue of proceeding with treatment of the spine without confirmation of malignancy arises. In such cases, it may be necessary to begin RT to the spine without a definitive diagnosis, but this must be done with the full understanding of the patient (and other members of the care team) that a diagnosis has not been established and that RT may preclude making a diagnosis, particularly in the setting of a radiosensitive tumor, e.g., lymphoma or germinoma. In such cases, it is often worthwhile to obtain a biopsy of the lesion before starting RT and, then, initiate RT while awaiting the results of that biopsy.

Treatment of spinal metastases may consist of conventional external-beam RT or SRS. Treatment of spinal metastases with external-beam RT has a long history and treatment may be begun very quickly, often within a few hours of the decision to treat. A variety of dosing schemes have been evaluated, ranging from a single 8 Gy fraction to twenty 2 Gy fractions. For bone metastases in general, there does not appear to be a significant difference in pain relief between the various regimens, with about one-third of patients exhibiting complete pain relief and the majority experiencing substantial decrease in pain following RT [67]. However, a prospective study of short- (one 8-Gy or five 4-Gy fractions) versus long-course (ten 3 Gy or twenty 2 fractions) spinal RT showed that the more protracted regimens were associated with a significantly reduced rate of recurrence [68]. This study showed no definite difference in functional outcome between the regimens. Note that many patients with spinal metastases have been previously treated with RT for thoracic or abdominal malignancies and have received some dose of radiation to the spine. Potentially, this increases the risk of radiation-induced myelopathy and it is essential to obtain and consider the history of prior RT before making a decision on the treatment modality and radiation dose.

In treatment of a metastasis to the osseous spine with SRS, the target is the portion of the vertebral body at risk with delivery of a purposely low dose of radiation to the spinal cord. Thus, SRS is especially useful when the spinal cord has previously received radiation. In comparison to conventional radiotherapy, SRS is a much more complex procedure, requiring specialized expertise, equipment and procedures [56]. While very high rates of palliation and freedom from recurrence [56, 58], along with low rates of radiation-induced myelopathy [69–71], have been reported, no randomized trial of SRS versus conventional RT in spinal metastases has been completed. The Radiation Therapy Oncology Group is currently conducting a randomized trial (RTOG 0618) comparing SRS versus conventional RT.

References

1. Black PM, Loeffler JS. Cancer of the nervous system. 2nd ed. Philadelphia: Lippincott Williams & Wilkins; 2005.
2. Halperin EC, Wazer DE, Perez CA. The discipline of radiation oncology. In: Halperin EC, Wazer DE, Paerez CA, et al., editors. Principle and practice of radiation oncology. 6th ed. Philadelphia: Lippincott Williams & Wilkins; 2013. p. 2–60.
3. Hall EJ, Giaccia AJ. Radiobiology for the radiologist. 7th ed. Philadelphia: Wolters Kluwer Health/Lippincott Williams & Wilkins; 2012.
4. Kirkpatrick JP, Milano MT, Constine LS, et al. Late effects and QUANTEC. In: Halperin EC, Wazer DE, Perez CA, et al., editors. Principles and practice of radiation oncology. 6th ed. Philadelphia: Lippincott Williams & Wilkens; 2013. p. 296–329.
5. Kirkpatrick JP, Yin FF, Sampson JH. Radiotherapy and radiosurgery for tumors of the central nervous system. Surg Oncol Clin N Am. 2013;22:445–61.
6. Barnett GH, Linskey ME, Adler JR, et al. Stereotactic radiosurgery – an organized neurosurgery-sanctioned definition. J Neurosurg. 2007;106:1–5.
7. Sperduto PW, Chao ST, Sneed PK, et al. Diagnosis-specific prognostic factors, indexes, and treatment outcomes for patients with newly diagnosed brain metastases: a multi-institutional analysis of 4,259 patients. Int J Radiat Oncol Biol Phys. 2010;77:655–61.

8. Mehta MP, Paleologos NA, Mikkelsen T, et al. The role of che-motherapy in the management of newly diagnosed brain metas-tases: a systematic review and evidence-based clinical practice guideline. J Neurooncol. 2010;96:71–83.

9. Mikkelsen T, Paleologos NA, Robinson PD, et al. The role of prophylactic anticonvulsants in the management of brain metas-tases: a systematic review and evidence-based clinical practice guideline. J Neurooncol. 2010;96:97–102.

10. Ryken TC, McDermott M, Robinson PD, et al. The role of ste-roids in the management of brain metastases: a systematic review and evidence-based clinical practice guideline. J Neurooncol. 2010;96:103–14.

11. Klein M, Heimans JJ, Aaronson NK, et al. Effect of radiotherapy and other treatment-related factors on mid-term to long-term cognitive sequelae in low-grade gliomas: a comparative study. Lancet. 2002;360:1361–8.

12. Douw L, Klein M, Fagel SS, et al. Cognitive and radiological effects of radiotherapy in patients with low-grade glioma: long-term follow-up. Lancet Neurol. 2009;8:810–8.

13. Tsao MN, Lloyd N, Wong RK, et al. Whole brain radiotherapy for the treatment of newly diagnosed multiple brain metastases. Cochrane Database Syst Rev. 2012;(4):CD003869.

14. Mintz AH, Kestle J, Rathbone MP, et al. A randomized trial to assess the efficacy of surgery in addition to radiotherapy in patients with a single cerebral metastasis. Cancer. 1996;78:1470–6.

15. Noordijk EM, Vecht CJ, Haaxma-Reiche H, et al. The choice of treatment of single brain metastasis should be based on extra-cranial tumor activity and age. Int J Radiat Oncol Biol Phys. 1994;29:711–7.

16. Patchell RA, Tibbs PA, Walsh JW, et al. A randomized trial of surgery in the treatment of single metastases to the brain. N Engl J Med. 1990;322:494–500.

17. Patchell RA, Tibbs PA, Regine WF, et al. Postoperative radio-therapy in the treatment of single metastases to the brain: a randomized trial. JAMA. 1998;280:1485–9.

18. Kocher M, Soffietti R, Abacioglu U, et al. Adjuvant whole-brain radiotherapy versus observation after radiosurgery or surgical resection of one to three cerebral metastases: results of the EORTC 22952–26001 study. J Clin Oncol. 2011;29:134–41.

19. Andrews DW, Scott CB, Sperduto PW, et al. Whole brain radia-tion therapy with or without stereotactic radiosurgery boost for patients with one to three brain metastases: phase III results of the RTOG 9508 randomised trial. Lancet. 2004;363:1665–72.

20. Sneed PK, Suh JH, Goetsch SJ, et al. A multi-institutional review of radiosurgery alone vs. radiosurgery with whole brain radiotherapy as the initial management of brain metastases. Int J Radiat Oncol Biol Phys. 2002;53:519–26.

21. Aoyama H, Shirato H, Tago M, et al. Stereotactic radiosurgery plus whole-brain radiation therapy vs stereotactic radiosurgery alone for treatment of brain metastases: a randomized controlled trial. JAMA. 2006;295:2483–91.

22. Aoyama H, Tago M, Kato N, et al. Neurocognitive function of patients with brain metastasis who received either whole brain radiotherapy plus stereotactic radiosurgery or radiosurgery alone. Int J Radiat Oncol Biol Phys. 2007;68:1388–95.

23. Chang EL, Wefel JS, Hess KR, et al. Neurocognition in patients with brain metastases treated with radiosurgery or radiosurgery plus whole-brain irradiation: a randomised controlled trial. Lancet Oncol. 2009;10:1037–44.

24. Soltys SG, Adler JR, Lipani JD, et al. Stereotactic radiosurgery of the postoperative resection cavity for brain metastases. Int J Radiat Oncol Biol Phys. 2008;70:187–93.

25. Choi CY, Chang SD, Gibbs IC, et al. Stereotactic radiosurgery of the postoperative resection cavity for brain metastases: prospective evaluation of target margin on tumor control. Int J Radiat Oncol Biol Phys. 2012;84:336–42.

26. Dolecek TA, Propp JM, Stroup NE, Kruchko C. CBTRUS statistical report: primary brain and central nervous system tumors diagnosed in the United States in 2005–2009. Neuro Oncol. 2012;14 Suppl 5:v1–49.

27. Ricard D, Idbaih A, Ducray F, et al. Primary brain tumours in adults. Lancet. 2012;379:1984–96.

28. Stummer W, van den Bent MJ, Westphal M. Cytoreductive surgery of glioblastoma as the key to successful adjuvant therapies: new arguments in an old discussion. Acta Neurochir (Wien). 2011;153:1211–8.

29. Laperriere NJ, Leung PM, McKenzie S, et al. Randomized study of brachytherapy in the initial management of patients with malignant astrocytoma. Int J Radiat Oncol Biol Phys. 1998;41:1005–11.

30. Walker MD, Alexander Jr E, Hunt WE, et al. Evaluation of BCNU and/or radiotherapy in the treatment of anaplastic gliomas. A cooperative clinical trial. J Neurosurg. 1978;49:333–43.

31. Bleehen NM, Stenning SP. A Medical Research Council trial of two radiotherapy doses in the treatment of grades 3 and 4

astrocytoma. The Medical Research Council Brain Tumour Working Party. Br J Cancer. 1991;64:769–74.

32. Walker MD, Strike TA, Sheline GE. An analysis of dose-effect relationship in the radiotherapy of malignant gliomas. Int J Radiat Oncol Biol Phys. 1979;5:1725–31.

33. Chang CH, Horton J, Schoenfeld D, et al. Comparison of postoperative radiotherapy and combined postoperative radiotherapy and chemotherapy in the multidisciplinary management of malignant gliomas. A joint Radiation Therapy Oncology Group and Eastern Cooperative Oncology Group study. Cancer. 1983;52:997–1007.

34. Nelson DF, Curran Jr WJ, Scott C, et al. Hyperfractionated radiation therapy and bis-chlorethyl nitrosourea in the treatment of malignant glioma–possible advantage observed at 72.0 Gy in 1.2 Gy B.I.D. fractions: report of the Radiation Therapy Oncology Group Protocol 8302. Int J Radiat Oncol Biol Phys. 1993;25: 193–207.

35. Selker RG, Shapiro WR, Burger P, et al. The Brain Tumor Cooperative Group NIH Trial 87–01: a randomized comparison of surgery, external radiotherapy, and carmustine versus surgery, interstitial radiotherapy boost, external radiation therapy, and carmustine. Neurosurgery. 2002;51:343–55; discussion 355–7.

36. Souhami L, Seiferheld W, Brachman D, et al. Randomized comparison of stereotactic radiosurgery followed by conventional radiotherapy with carmustine to conventional radiotherapy with carmustine for patients with glioblastoma multiforme: report of Radiation Therapy Oncology Group 93–05 protocol. Int J Radiat Oncol Biol Phys. 2004;60:853–60.

37. Shih HA. Oncology scan – high-grade gliomas. Int J Radiat Oncol Biol Phys. 2013;85:283–5.

38. Hochberg FH, Pruitt A. Assumptions in the radiotherapy of glioblastoma. Neurology. 1980;30:907–11.

39. Shapiro WR, Young DF. Treatment of malignant glioma. A controlled study of chemotherapy and irradiation. Arch Neurol. 1976;33:494–50.

40. Wallner KE, Galicich JH, Krol G, et al. Patterns of failure following treatment for glioblastoma multiforme and anaplastic astrocytoma. Int J Radiat Oncol Biol Phys. 1989;16:1405–9.

41. Fine HA, Dear KB, Loeffler JS, et al. Meta-analysis of radiation therapy with and without adjuvant chemotherapy for malignant gliomas in adults. Cancer. 1993;71:2585–97.

42. Stewart LA. Chemotherapy in adult high-grade glioma: a systematic review and meta-analysis of individual patient data from 12 randomised trials. Lancet. 2002;359:1011–8.
43. Stupp R, Hegi ME, Mason WP, et al. Effects of radiotherapy with concomitant and adjuvant temozolomide versus radiotherapy alone on survival in glioblastoma in a randomised phase III study: 5-year analysis of the EORTC-NCIC trial. Lancet Oncol. 2009;10:459–66.
44. Cohen MH, Shen YL, Keegan P, et al. FDA drug approval summary: bevacizumab (Avastin) as treatment of recurrent glioblastoma multiforme. Oncologist. 2009;14:1131–8.
45. Kreisl TN, Kim L, Moore K, et al. Phase II trial of single-agent bevacizumab followed by bevacizumab plus irinotecan at tumor progression in recurrent glioblastoma. J Clin Oncol. 2009;27:740–5.
46. Vredenburgh JJ, Desjardins A, Herndon 2nd JE, et al. Phase II trial of bevacizumab and irinotecan in recurrent malignant glioma. Clin Cancer Res. 2007;13:1253–9.
47. Fogh SE, Andrews DW, Glass J, et al. Hypofractionated stereotactic radiation therapy: an effective therapy for recurrent high-grade gliomas. J Clin Oncol. 2010;28:3048–53.
48. Cabrera AR, Cuneo KC, Desjardins A, et al. Concurrent stereotactic radiosurgery and bevacizumab in recurrent malignant gliomas: a prospective trial. Int J Radiat Oncol Biol Phys. 2013;86:873–9.
49. Cuneo KC, Vredenburgh JJ, Sampson JH, et al. Safety and efficacy of stereotactic radiosurgery and adjuvant bevacizumab in patients with recurrent malignant gliomas. Int J Radiat Oncol Biol Phys. 2012;82:2018–24.
50. Gutin PH, Iwamoto FM, Beal K, et al. Safety and efficacy of bevacizumab with hypofractionated stereotactic irradiation for recurrent malignant gliomas. Int J Radiat Oncol Biol Phys. 2009;75:156–63.
51. Ma L, Sahgal A, Cozzi L, et al. Apparatus-dependent dosimetric differences in spine stereotactic body radiotherapy. Technol Cancer Res Treat. 2010;9:563–74.
52. Nelson JW, Yoo DS, Sampson JH, et al. Stereotactic body radiotherapy for lesions of the spine and paraspinal regions. Int J Radiat Oncol Biol Phys. 2009;73:1369–75.
53. Wu QJ, Wang Z, Kirkpatrick JP, et al. Impact of collimator leaf width and treatment technique on stereotactic radiosurgery and radiotherapy plans for intra- and extracranial lesions. Radiat Oncol. 2009;4:3.

54. Wu QJ, Yoo S, Kirkpatrick JP, et al. Volumetric arc intensity-modulated therapy for spine body radiotherapy: comparison with static intensity-modulated treatment. Int J Radiat Oncol Biol Phys. 2009;75:1596–604.

55. Sahgal A, Bilsky M, Chang EL, et al. Stereotactic body radio-therapy for spinal metastases: current status, with a focus on its application in the postoperative patient. J Neurosurg Spine. 2011;14:151–66.

56. Sahgal A, Larson DA, Chang EL. Stereotactic body radiosurgery for spinal metastases: a critical review. Int J Radiat Oncol Biol Phys. 2008;71:652–65.

57. Ahmed KA, Stauder MC, Miller RC, et al. Stereotactic body radiation therapy in spinal metastases. Int J Radiat Oncol Biol Phys. 2012;82:e803–9.

58. Hall WA, Stapleford LJ, Hadjipanayis CG, et al. Stereotactic body radiosurgery for spinal metastatic disease: an evidence-based review. Int J Surg Oncol. 2011;2011:979214.

59. Sciubba DM, Petteys RJ, Dekutoski MB, et al. Diagnosis and management of metastatic spine disease. A review. J Neurosurg Spine. 2010;13:94–108.

60. Bach F, Larsen BH, Rohde K, et al. Metastatic spinal cord compression. Occurrence, symptoms, clinical presentations and prognosis in 398 patients with spinal cord compression. Acta Neurochir (Wien). 1990;107:37–43.

61. Helweg-Larsen S, Sorensen PS. Symptoms and signs in metastatic spinal cord compression: a study of progression from first symptom until diagnosis in 153 patients. Eur J Cancer. 1994;30A:396–8.

62. Loblaw DA, Mitera G, Ford M, et al. A 2011 updated systematic review and clinical practice guideline for the management of malignant extradural spinal cord compression. Int J Radiat Oncol Biol Phys. 2012;84:312–7.

63. Rades D, Blach M, Nerreter V, et al. Metastatic spinal cord compression. Influence of time between onset of motoric deficits and start of irradiation on therapeutic effect. Strahlenther Onkol. 1999;175:378–81.

64. Rades D, Heidenreich F, Karstens JH. Final results of a prospective study of the prognostic value of the time to develop motor deficits before irradiation in metastatic spinal cord compression. Int J Radiat Oncol Biol Phys. 2002;53:975–9.

65. Patchell RA, Tibbs PA, Regine WF, et al. Direct decompressive surgical resection in the treatment of spinal cord compression

caused by metastatic cancer: a randomised trial. Lancet. 2005;366:643–8.

66. Rades D, Huttenlocher S, Dunst J, et al. Matched pair analysis comparing surgery followed by radiotherapy and radiotherapy alone for metastatic spinal cord compression. J Clin Oncol. 2010;28:3597–604.

67. Lutz S, Berk L, Chang E, et al. Palliative radiotherapy for bone metastases: an ASTRO evidence-based guideline. Int J Radiat Oncol Biol Phys. 2011;79:965–76.

68. Rades D, Lange M, Veninga T, et al. Final results of a prospective study comparing the local control of short-course and long-course radiotherapy for metastatic spinal cord compression. Int J Radiat Oncol Biol Phys. 2011;79:524–30.

69. Kirkpatrick JP, van der Kogel AJ, Schultheiss TE. Radiation dose-volume effects in the spinal cord. Int J Radiat Oncol Biol Phys. 2010;76:S42–9.

70. Sahgal A, Ma L, Gibbs I, et al. Spinal cord tolerance for stereotactic body radiotherapy. Int J Radiat Oncol Biol Phys. 2010;77:548–53.

71. Sahgal A, Weinberg V, Ma L, et al. Probabilities of radiation myelopathy specific to stereotactic body radiation therapy to guide safe practice. Int J Radiat Oncol Biol Phys. 2013;85: 341–7.

Chapter 12
Peripheral Nerve Problems: An Overview for Patients and Their Family Members

Harjus S. Birk, Tene Cage, and Michel Kliot

Peripheral nerves enter and exit the brain, via cranial nerves, and the spinal cord, via spinal nerves. Peripheral nerves which form the Peripheral Nervous System (PNS) transmit sensory information (such as touch, pain and temperature) into the Central Nervous System (CNS) and exert control over muscles which allows one to perform voluntary movements and actions (such as speaking, eating, writing, typing and playing sports). Damage to peripheral nerves therefore can result in altered or loss of sensation and weakness or paralysis. The pattern of altered sensation and strength depends upon the specific peripheral nerve(s) involved as well as the type and location of peripheral nerve problem.

H.S. Birk
School of Medicine, University of California,
San Francisco, CA, USA

T. Cage
Department of Neurosurgery, University of California,
San Francisco, CA, USA

M. Kliot, MD (✉)
Department of Neurosurgery, University of Northwestern Feinberg School of Medicine,
676 North St. Clair Street, Suite 2210, Chicago 60611, IL, USA
e-mail: michelkliot@gmail.com

A. Agrawal, G. Britz (eds.), *Comprehensive Guide to Neurosurgical Conditions*, DOI 10.1007/978-3-319-06566-3_12,
© Springer International Publishing Switzerland 2015

Although some peripheral nerves are sensory and only convey sensation while others are motor and only control movement, the majority of peripheral nerves are mixed and mediate both sensory and motor function.

In this chapter, we will discuss the most common peripheral nerve problems such as nerve entrapment syndromes, traumatic nerve injuries, and masses arising from nerves such as tumors. We will begin each section by first discussing how the problem presents with clinical symptoms and findings. We will then discuss the underlying pathology and diagnostic studies used to diagnose the specific problem, and finally we will analyze the treatment options which include physical therapy, careful observation, and, when warranted, surgical intervention. It is our hope that in so doing we can educate patients and their family so that they are well informed when seeking and undergoing treatment for a wide variety of peripheral nerve problems.

Peripheral Nerve Entrapment Syndromes

When under pressure or stretched, peripheral nerve fibers, also known as axons, lose their insulation know as myelin that is produced by Schwann cells. This demyelination of the nerve results in a decrease in the speed of conduction of nerve impulses that can lead to alterations in sensation and function. If the compression and stretch is severe or prolonged then nerve fibers, also known as axons, actually begin to die which can lead to muscle wasting also known as atrophy. The goal of early diagnosis is to catch nerve entrapment syndromes in the early phase when medical therapy is more effective. In later stages, especially if the loss of axons has occurred, surgery is usually required for recovery to occur.

What follows is a clinical description of nerve entrapment syndromes. Non-surgical treatment involves avoidance of painful postures or movements, use of ergonomic devices where appropriate, non-steroidal medication and avoidance of narcotic drugs particularly for long-term use, local injection of steroid and/or local anesthetic to help confirm the diagnosis and provide symptom relief that is usually temporary, and physical therapy sometimes supplemented with massage therapy where appropriate. Surgical decompression of the nerve should be considered when these measures fail and its success is increased when there is electrodiagnostic evidence on electromyographic (EMG) and nerve conduction velocity (NCV) studies, which help confirm the diagnosis.

Carpal Tunnel Syndrome

Carpal Tunnel Syndrome (CTS) is due to the compression of the median nerve within a space called the carpal tunnel. It is believed that the prevalence of CTS in the general population is 2–3 %. CTS is more common in men than women and most often occurs between the ages of 40 and 60. Certain conditions that predispose to the development of CTS include pregnancy with resolution of hand symptoms following delivery, as well as diabetes, acromegaly, and hypothyroidism.

The incidence of CTS is more common in people practicing certain professions that involve long periods of performing repetitive hand maneuvers. For example, people who work especially cold environments, including meat and fish packing workers, as well as typists, key board operators, musicians, and assembly line workers, are more likely to develop carpal tunnel syndrome (Allieu et al.).

Classic symptoms of carpal tunnel syndrome include wrist pain and numbness in the thumb, index, and middle fingers. Although pain in the forearm and even the upper arm may occur with CTS, pain in the neck is rare and suggests a problem at the level of the spine. Tapping or applying direct pressure over the carpal tunnel space in the palm and the wrist, as well as either excessive flexion or extension of the hand across the wrist, may make the wrist pain and finger numbness worse, so it is best to avoid such postures.

In addition to clinical symptoms and findings, the diagnosis is strengthened when confirmed by electrodiagnostic studies such as nerve conduction velocity (NVC) studies showing slowed conduction of the median nerve across the carpal tunnel and an electromyogram (EMG) showing abnormalities in the thenar muscles of the hand in more severe cases. In some instances, an MRI of the carpal tunnel may be useful in visualizing abnormalities such as the rare presence of cysts or tumors.

Medical therapy for carpal tunnel syndrome consists of a combination of avoiding hand activities that worsen the symptoms of wrist pain and finger numbness (e.g., repetitive movements such as typing), as well as appropriate ergonomic changes aimed at keeping the wrist in a neutral position. Wrist splinting and formal hand therapy should be tried initially for at least a period of several weeks. The injection of steroids into the carpal tunnel space can also provide temporary relief of symptoms as well as help confirm the diagnosis of CTS. Furthermore, non-steroidal anti-inflammatory drugs can also be used to treat the symptoms of carpal tunnel syndrome, but narcotic medications should be avoided. These medical measures in many cases are effective in improving the symptoms of patients with mild and moderate CTS (i.e., intermittent or continuous symptoms respectively but no clinical or EMG evidence of axonal loss).

In patients with severe CTS (i.e. those with evidence of axonal loss) or those who fail the medical measures described above, surgical decompression of the median nerve should be considered. Extensive reviews of the literature have found that surgery is more effective than splinting for patients with carpal tunnel syndrome (Jarvik et al.). For example, those patients who do undergo surgery can expect an 80–90 % chance of improvement.

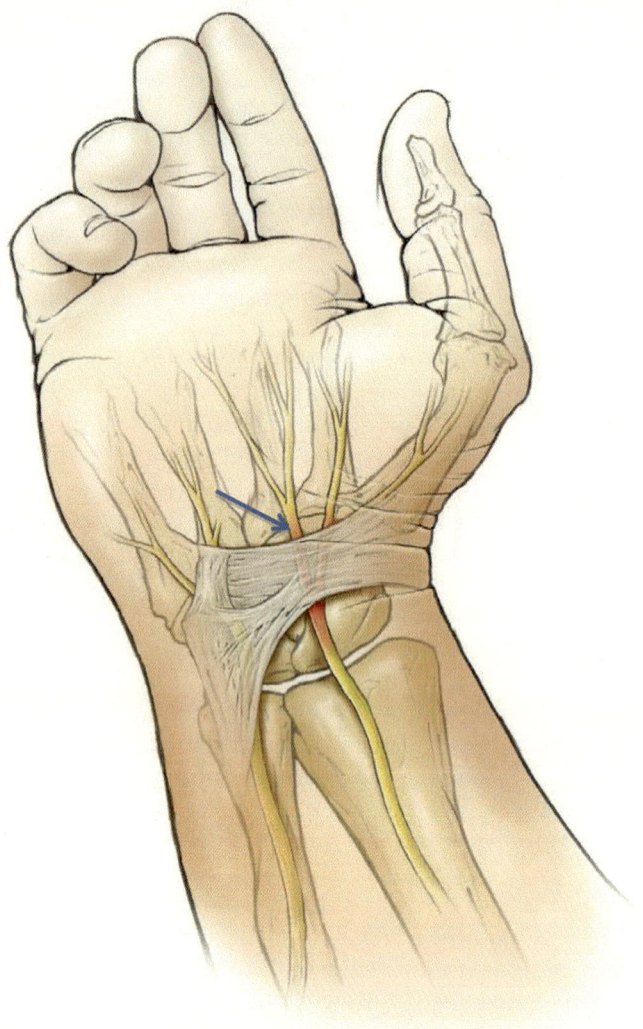

FIGURE 12.1 Schematic drawing showing median nerve compressed (*red zone*) within the carpal tunnel

Ulnar Nerve Entrapment Within the Cubital Tunnel of the Elbow

The ulnar nerve can become compressed across the elbow within the cubital tunnel, a condition known as cubital tunnel syndrome. It is the second most common nerve entrapment syndrome after CTS. Patients complain of numbness and tingling usually in the ring and little fingers, often exacerbated when the arm is fully flexed across the elbow. Initial treatment involves avoiding direct pressure to the nerve, sometimes facilitated by using an elbow pad, as well as avoiding postures that exacerbate the symptoms, such as using a splint across the elbow when sleeping to keep the arm from flexing. If these measures fail, surgical decompression of the nerve across the elbow can be performed (Allagui et al.). In some usually more severe cases, the ulnar nerve is not only decompressed but also moved or transposed slightly

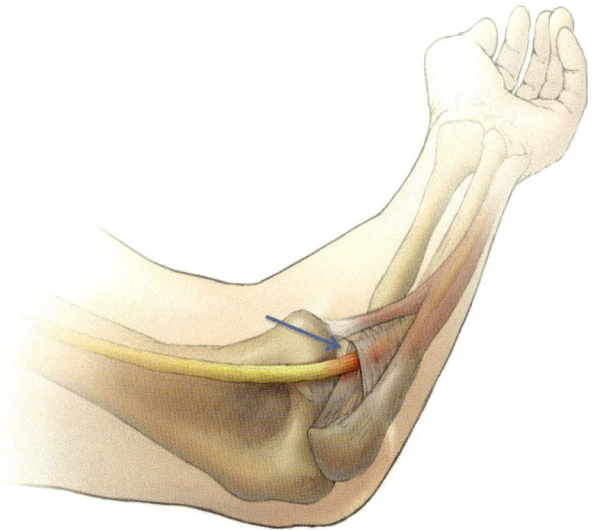

FIGURE 12.2 Schematic drawing showing ulnar nerve becoming compressed (*red zone*) as it enters the cubital tunnel across the elbow

to a more lateral and protected location where its distance across the elbow is shorter, thereby making it less prone to being stretched and put under tension.

Thoracic Outlet Syndrome

Thoracic Outlet Sundrome (TOS) occurs when the nerves in the neck, also known as the brachial plexus (called neurogenic TOS), or adjacent large blood vessels such as the subclavian artery (called vascular TOS) become compressed by adjacent bone, connective tissue, and/or muscular tissue. TOS causes pain in the neck and the shoulder that can radiate down the arm into the hand and fingers, as well as numbness and weakness in more advanced cases. The lower portion of the brachial plexus supplying the hand muscles, also known as the lower trunk, is most often involved. These symptoms and findings are usually made worse with arm abduction at the shoulder such as when the patient raises or uses his hand above shoulder level. An extra cervical rib or enlarged transverse process of the spine at the C7/T1 level predisposes patients to developing this syndrome. In addition to physical therapy aimed at stretching out the scalene muscles that may lessen nerve compression, image guided injection of Botox into the scalene muscles which causes reversible paralysis may be helpful both to diagnose and treat this condition. In cases, where these treatments fail, a surgical decompression may be helpful.

Pronator Teres Syndrome

Median nerve compression in the proximal forearm is referred to as pronator teres syndrome. It is rare compared to carpal tunnel syndrome and causes pain in the forearm as well as weakness in flexing the thumb and index finger. Patients with pronator teres syndrome usually have difficulty turning their palm downwards (pronation) against resistance because this action is very painful. Treatment of pronator teres syndrome includes avoidance of painful movements, as well as steroid injections and massage therapy, and, when these measures fail, surgical decompression of the nerve (Zancolli et al.). The diagnosis is confirmed with either electro diagnostic or imaging studies.

Radial Tunnel Syndrome

Radial Tunnel Syndrome is due to compression of the radial nerve in the proximal forearm which causes pain when turning the palm up (supination) against resistance. Treatment of this condition involves avoidance of exacerbating movements as well as non-steroidal anti-inflammatory drugs, massage therapy, and surgery when conservative measures fail (Naam et al.).

Guyon's Canal Syndrome

Guyon's Canal Syndrome results when the ulnar nerve becomes trapped in a space called the Guyon's canal in the hand. Patients with this syndrome initially complain of a sensation of pins and needles in the ring and pinky fingers and may progress to a reduction in hand function. Guyon's canal syndrome is very commonly seen in cyclists who experience a lot of pressure against the palm area when gripping the handlebars. Treatment for this syndrome includes avoidance of exacerbating postures as well as non-steroidal anti-inflammatory drugs, massage therapy, and injection of steroids in the canal. When these therapeutic measures fail, surgical decompression can be performed.

Pyriformis Syndrome

Pyriformis Syndrome is characterized by compression of the sciatic nerve by the overlying pyriformis muscle which may fibrose, located deep in the buttock. Patients with this syndrome will present with deep buttock pain and discomfort, and often pain

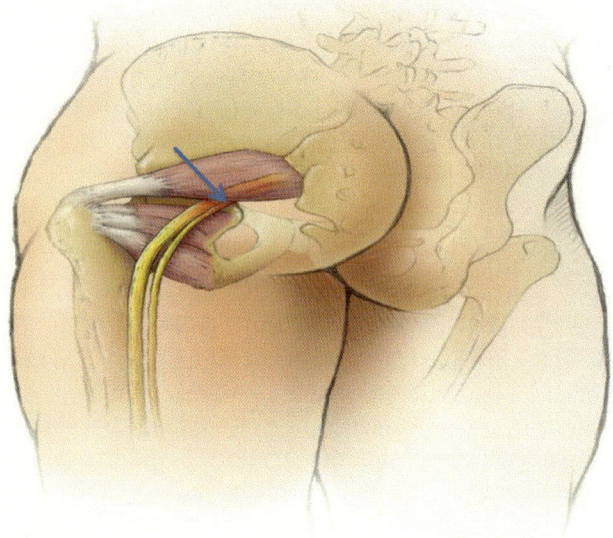

FIGURE 12.3 Schematic drawing showing sciatic nerve compressed (*red zone*) by overlying pyriformis muscle in the buttock after exiting the sciatic notch

radiating down the posterior thigh and lower leg (sciatica), exacerbated by pressure on the buttock such as when sitting for long periods of time. Treatment of this condition involves physical therapy directed at stretching out the pyriformis muscle. As in TOS, image guided injection of Botox into the pyriformis muscle combined with physical therapy may be useful to both diagnose and treat this condition. If these measures fail, a surgical decompression in which the pyriformis muscle is cut may prove helpful.

Meralgia Paresthetica

Meralgia Paresthetica describes a pain and/or numbness along the antero–lateral thigh that is caused by compression of the lateral femoral cutaneous nerve as it exits the pelvis and enters the inguinal canal. Treatment of meralgia paresthetica involves non-steroidal anti-inflammatory drugs, massage therapy, and, when the above measures fail, surgery in which the nerve is either decompressed or actually cut.

Tarsal Tunnel Syndrome

Tarsal Tunnel Syndrome is a painful foot condition caused by compression of the tibial nerve as it passes through a space along the medial ankle called the tarsal tunnel. Numbness and pain usually involves the sole of the foot (Imai et al.). Treatment of this condition includes steroid injections, massage therapy, and in some cases surgery to decompress the tibial nerve (Maniker et al.).

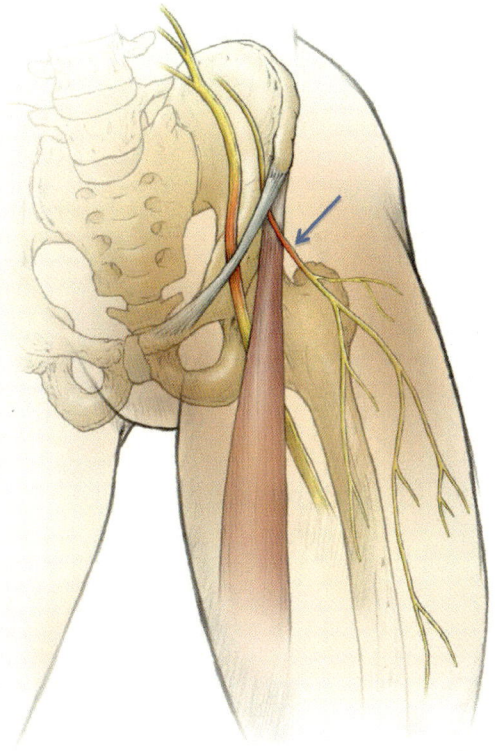

FIGURE 12.4 Schematic diagram showing left lateral femoral cutaneous nerve compressed as it passes through the inguinal ligament (*red zone*)

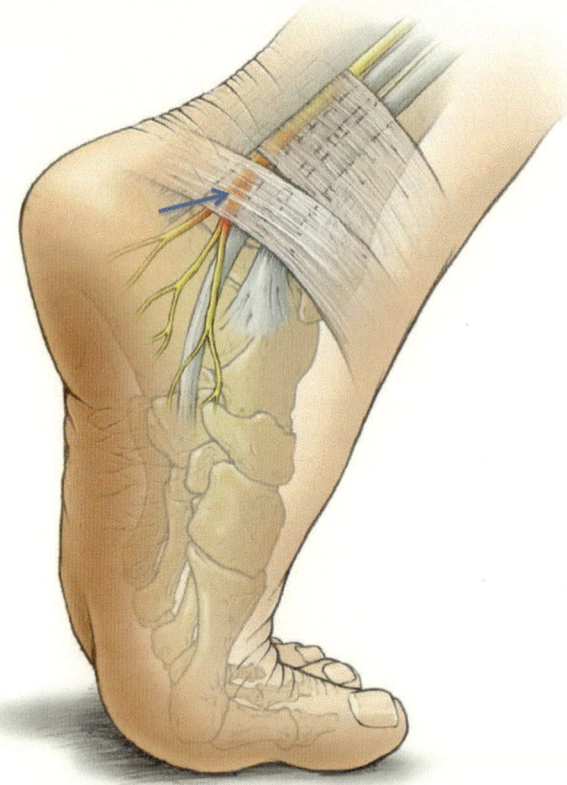

FIGURE 12.5 Schematic drawing showing compression of the tibial nerve (*red zone*) within the tarsal tunnel

Peroneal Entrapment at the Fibular Head

When the peroneal nerve becomes compressed in the lower leg as it passes around the fibular head it may cause tingling along the top of the foot as well as weakness in dorsiflexing (taking one's foot off the gas pedal) the foot and toes. Treatment of this condition involves avoidance of exacerbating movements, such as deep knee bends, as well as non-steroidal anti-inflammatory drugs and surgical decompression of the nerve when conservative measures are not effective in alleviating symptoms.

Traumatic Nerve Injuries

The ability to recover from traumatic peripheral nerve injuries depends on how severe the injury is. Peripheral nerve injuries can be grouped into three categories: mild, moderate, and severe (Birch et al.).

Mild injuries cause damage primarily to the supporting cells, called Schwann cells, that insulate the nerve fiber or axons with myelin. Mild injuries can be diagnosed with nerve conduction studies which show slowing or no conduction of nerve impulses across the damaged segment of demyelinated nerve. Since the axons remain intact, stimulation of the nerve distal to the demyelinated segment produces a nerve impulse and muscle contraction in the case of a motor nerve. Such injuries can recover on their own over a period of weeks to months and often result in full restoration of function.

In a moderate injury, the nerve fiber or axon is damaged to the point where it degenerates and no longer transmits an electrical impulse on nerve conduction studies. The EMG shows characteristic changes that develop in muscle when deprived of their nerve supply. However, the cellular and molecular structure and architecture around the axons is preserved, thereby allowing nerve fibers to slowly grow or regenerate and regain their ability to transmit electrical nerve signals. With moderate injuries, nerve fibers regenerate at a rate of about 1 in. per month and so the degree and timing of recovery depends on the distance axons must regenerate to reach their sensory or motor targets, as well as the complexity of the nerve pathways that they must navigate.

Severe nerve injuries involve either actual cutting of a nerve or damage that produces so much of a scar within the nerve that the regeneration of nerve fibers is blocked.

In severe nerve injuries, the loss of function is therefore permanent unless a surgical repair is performed. Immediately after a traumatic injury, the nerve conduction and EMG findings will be similar for both a moderate and severe nerve injury. In a moderate injury as axonal regeneration occurs, the nerve conduction and EMG findings will improve as recovery of functions occurs. Since axonal regeneration cannot occur in a severe injury, the nerve conduction and EMG findings will not improve over time and there will be no recovery of function (Grant et al.).

In severe injuries where the nerve has been completely cut but there is not a large gap, the two ends can be surgically trimmed and sutured back together. Nerve repair may involve direct repair of the damaged nerve, or use of a graft or tube (usually made from a bioabsorbable material such as collagen) when the two nerve ends cannot be brought together without causing tension. A nerve graft is usually a sensory nerve harvested from another part of the body, such as the sural nerve in the lower leg, whose sacrifice does not produce a significant functional deficit. Specially processed human cadaveric nerve grafts can also be used. The nerve graft or the tube serves as a bridge which allows regenerating nerve fibers to grow from the proximal nerve stump through the distal nerve segment once the graft is in place. Nerve repair is usually performed by the surgeon using magnification provided by special eye glasses or a miscroscope. Special electrophysiological nerve stimulation and recording techniques are often used to help identify and distinguish functioning from non-functioning nerve and thereby help avoid damage to working nerve fibers. A period of reduced movement for two weeks of the limb involved in a nerve repair is recommended after surgery to avoid disrupting the nerve repair site (Russell et al.).

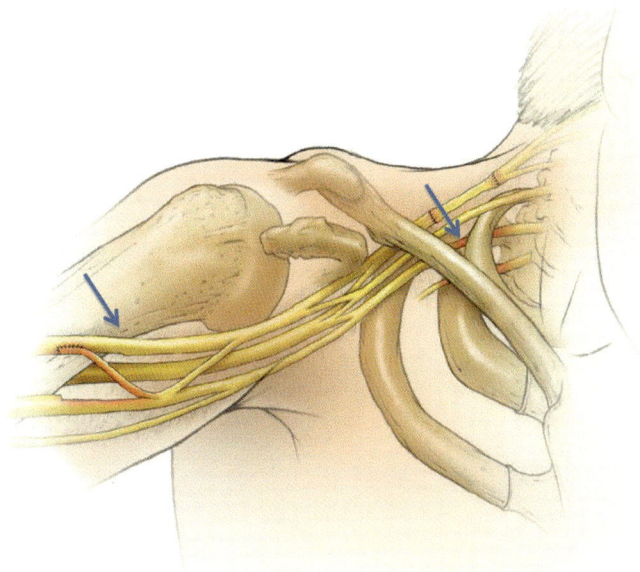

Figure 12.6 Schematic drawing showing nerve graft repair (**a**) of right brachial plexus in the neck as well as nerve repair not using a graft (**b**) in the upper arm

Masses

The majority of peripheral nerve masses are Schwannomas or Neurofibromas. Schwannomas are benign tumors affecting Schwann cells, which form the myelin around axons that acts as insulation and helps to speed up nerve conduction. Schwannomas may involve any nerve. Neurofibromas are often seen in patients with Neurofibromatosis (NF) of which there are several types. Patients with NF Type 1 have masses involving their peripheral nerve primarily whereas patients with NF Type 2 have neurofibromas involving their 8th cranial nerve arising from the brain as well. The symptoms and findings caused by these masses depend upon the nerves from which they arise and can include pain, numbness, weakness, and tingling.

Both schwannomas and neurofibromas may stop growing for long periods of time and can be therefore observed with

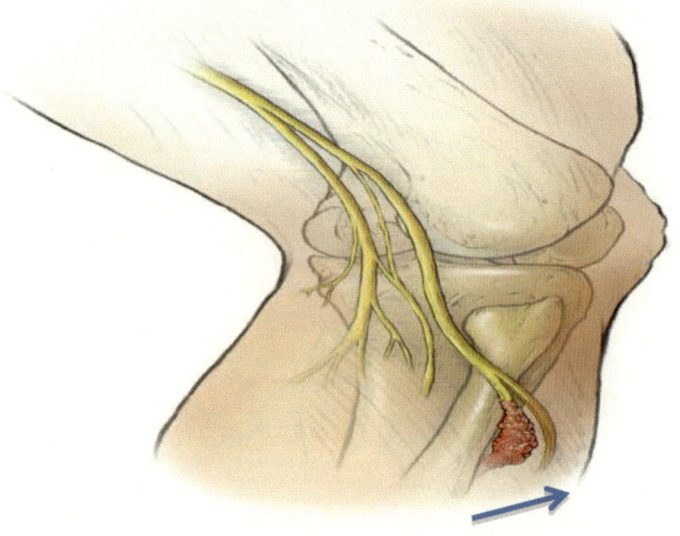

FIGURE 12.7 Schematic drawing showing a nerve tumor arising from one of the right peroneal nerve branches in the lower leg

follow-up exams and imaging studies such as MRI, ultrasound, and CT scans to pinpoint the location and size of the tumor. However, some of these masses continue to grow and/or become symptomatic. It is these tumors that require surgery both to make a definitive diagnosis and to remove the tumor whenever possible while trying to spare function. These tumors are best dealt with at medical centers with experience and special expertise that includes the ability to monitor sensory and motor nerve function during surgery. A few of these tumors may become malignant and require a more aggressive approach that involves not only surgery but also the administration of chemotherapy and radiation therapy.

Other masses that involve peripheral nerve include ganglion cysts which often involve the peroneal nerve in the lower leg near the fibular head. These cysts are benign and can be treated with surgery aimed at decompressing the cyst and cutting the nerve branch arising from the joint that provides a conduit for the movement of gelatinous joint fluid into the nerve.

References

1. Allagui M. Ulnar nerve compression at the elbow and hetero-topic ossification. Neurosurgery. 2010;56(4):340–343.
2. Allieu Y, MacKinnon S. Nerve compression syndromes of the upper limb. London: Martin Dunitz; 2002.
3. Birch R. Peripheral nerve injuries: a clinical guide. London: Springer; 2013.
4. Grant G, Goodkin R, Michel K. Evaluation and surgical management of peripheral nerve problems. Neurosurgery. 1999; 44(4):825–39.
5. Imai K. Tarsal tunnel syndrome. Foot Ank. Int. 2013;34(3):439–444.
6. Jarvik JG. MR neuroimaging in a prospective cohort of patients with suspected carpal tunnel syndrome. Neurology. 2002;11: 1597–1602.
7. Maniker A. Operative exposures in peripheral nerve surgery. New York: Thieme; 2004.
8. Naam NH. Radial tunnel syndrome. Plan & Reconstruc Surg. 2012;43(4):529–536.
9. Russell S. Examination of peripheral nerve injuries: an anatomical approach. New York: Thieme; 2006.
10. Zancolli ER, Penotto CJ. New mini-invasive decompression for pronatorteres syndrome. J Hand Surg Am. 2012;37(8):1706–1710.

Chapter 13
Rehabilitation of Neurosurgical Conditions

Teresa Kaldis and Purvi Desai

The Rehab Team

A comprehensive team of rehabilitation professionals are available to assist in the care and recovery of the patient's neurosurgical condition. Neurological conditions affect the brain, spine or both. The patient may benefit from evaluation from one or from many of the members of the rehab team below.

Neurosurgeon identifies the primary neurological issue and recommends a treatment plan. The neurosurgeon will decide precautions or restrictions for the patient and determine how long they need to be followed.

Physiatrist or Physical Medicine and Rehabilitation (Rehab doctor) specializes in evaluation of a person's functional and mobility status and makes recommendations for

T. Kaldis, MD, (✉)
Methodist Rehabilitation Associates,
Houston Methodist Hospital, 6560 Fannin,
Suite 1878, Houston, TX 77030, USA
e-mail: tkaldis@houstonmethodist.org

P. Desai, MD
Department of Physical Medicine and Rehabilitation,
Houston Methodist Hospital, 6560 Fannin, Suite 1878,
Houston, TX 77030, USA
e-mail: pndesai@tmhs.org

A. Agrawal, G. Britz (eds.), *Comprehensive Guide to Neurosurgical Conditions*, DOI 10.1007/978-3-319-06566-3_13,
© Springer International Publishing Switzerland 2015

various therapy services for recovery from a neurosurgical condition. They will monitor the progress in therapy, discuss with the team and make changes to the program as needed. They can prescribe medications and/or non-medicine treatments such as cold, heat, electrical stimulation or bracing.

Physical therapist addresses issues with mobility such as getting in and out of bed, standing, walking and climbing stairs. They help improve strength and balance and assess the need for a gait device such as a cane, walker or wheelchair.

Occupational therapist addresses the patient's ability to perform activities of daily living like grooming, dressing, toileting, and household task. They also assess the patient's ability to perform higher level tasks like driving, cooking, returning to work or other challenging tasks. They assess how vision, hearing, and thinking skills impact the patient's ability to do a certain task.

Speech language pathologist assesses voice for effective communication, safe swallowing, speech, cognitive and language skills. They address recommendations for a safe diet if swallowing muscles are affected. They will administer tests to identify issues with cognitive function and will provide treatment.

Neuropsychologist assesses neurocognitive function and can administer a more in-depth testing of cognitive, language and emotional skills. They make recommendations for patients and families for recovering from and coping with a neurological condition. They may also make recommendations to the rehab team about strategies to enhance performance.

Rehab nurse specializes in teaching and educating for neurological conditions with emphasis on bladder, bowel, skin, and medication management.

Social worker seeks to improve the quality of life and well-being by helping the individuals reach their full potential in their environment.

Case manager assists in the collaborative process of assessment, planning, facilitation, care coordination, and evaluation of healthcare needs and benefits.

Pharmacist educates the patient and their family on medication interaction and side effects.

Vocational counselor assists individuals whose health changes affect their ability to work and educates them on ways to adapt or change vocations.

Levels of Care

During treatment and recovery, the patient may transition through various levels of hospital care before eventually completing treatment as an outpatient, or they may be treated only in an outpatient setting. It is common for patients to transition to various rehabilitation locations (post-acute settings) during their recovery. An evaluation will occur in the Neuro-Intensive Care Unit (NICU) or Neurosurgical (NS) floor to assess and recommend the best steps based on the patient's medical and therapy needs. The case manager will then make the referral to the appropriate post-acute facility. The case manager will assist with the insurance approval process for post-acute services.

NICU depending on the injury or surgery you may require intensive care unit (ICU) level care

Neurosurgical floor specializes in post-op care of NS conditions

Acute inpatient rehab specializes in hospital care with focus on intensive therapy (3 h per day) and medical support

Skilled nursing facility (SNF) hospital level care that provides post-acute services including nursing support, nursing assistant and therapy services with less intense medical support

Long term acute care (LTAC) hospital level care that provides intense medical support by a physician with multiple consultants, nursing support and therapy services

Home Health Services provided at home for home-bound patients including nursing visits, wound care and therapy services

Outpatient therapy services provided at an outpatient location for physical, occupational and speech therapy. A person can receive services from single or multiple disciplines.

Home exercise program once the patient has been instructed on proper exercises, restrictions and precautions by their doctor and/or therapist they will perform these routines on their own.

Depending on individual needs, therapy may begin in the hospital and then transition to home or outpatient or you may begin in outpatient.

Rehab After Brain and Spinal Conditions

Brain

There are many factors that contribute to a rehabilitation program after an injury to or surgery on the brain. The team will help individualize each program and may include some or all of the professionals and services listed above. If the neurosurgeon removes part of the skull (skull flap), the patient may be required to wear a helmet to protect the brain until the bone flap can be replaced. In addition to possible physical difficulties with mobility, the patient may also have trouble with thinking, processing and executive dysfunction. Your team may recommend in-depth testing with a neuropsychologist to assess strengths and weaknesses to help plan rehabilitation needs and programs.

Spinal

There are many factors that contribute to a rehabilitation program after an injury to or surgery on the spine. The team will help individualize each program and may include some or all the professionals and services listed above. The neurosurgeon may want the patient to follow spinal precautions and perhaps wear a back brace for a period of time after the injury or surgery. The brace may have to be worn all of the time or only when upright or walking.

The surgeon will determine what restrictions or precautions the patient needs to follow after the procedure. Most of these limitations will be short-term to be followed for weeks, perhaps months. The rehab team will help the patient learn, adapt and incorporate these restrictions into daily life and into exercise program.

Symptoms

Neurosurgical diagnoses can lead to problems in the central and peripheral nervous system (CNS and PNS) involving the brain, spine, spinal cord or nerves. Depending on the location of the problem, the patient may experience a wide variety of symptoms.

Weakness of arms or legs
Difficulty walking (gait disturbance)
Difficulty talking or understanding
Difficulty swallowing
Change in mood/behavior
Dizziness
Confusion
Visual changes
Hearing changes
Decreased attention/concentration
Difficulty with short-term memory
Fatigue
Spasticity

Many of these symptoms or deficits benefit from treatment of a rehab specialist and improve with time. In consultation with the rehab team, there will be short- and long-term goals identified and an individual treatment plan recommended. They will help identify areas of strength and weakness as the patient strives to achieve maximal functional recovery.

Rehab Treatment Plan

Rehabilitation Program

A rehabilitation program will begin once the physician clears the patient to begin activities. This program may include physical therapy to work on gait/balance/transfer training and strengthening, occupational therapy to assist with independence with Activities of Daily Living (ADLs) and strengthening, and speech therapy to work on cognitive and/ or swallowing therapies. If the patient has significant weakness of key muscle groups, the therapist may begin functional electrical stimulation (FES) whereby small electrical impulses are delivered to motor nerves resulting in contraction of the muscle.

Pain Control

Pain is to be expected after any surgical intervention. When it interferes with the patient's ability to do out-of-bed activities or with sleep, changes may need to be made to the regimen. Post operatively, a patient may be placed on a Patient Controlled Analgesia (PCA) pump which allows the patient control over narcotic administration by pushing a button to deliver the medication straight into an IV. Within the first few days, the PCA will be weaned off and transitioned to oral versus IV narcotics. In addition, muscle relaxants are utilized in patients with muscle spasms in addition to ice or heat and topical patches/creams. Neuropathic (nerve related) pain can develop where nerves are affected causing tingling, burning or sharp shooting pains. The treatment can include oral agents (gabapentin, Lyrica, Cymbalta, etc.) or Transcutaneous Electrical Nerve Stimulation (TENS). TENS units work by sending small electrical impulses across the surface of the skin and nerve strands to prevent the pain signals from reaching the brain.

Bracing

For patients who undergo spinal surgery or who sustain an injury to the spine, the surgeon may recommend placing the patient in a neck or back brace for 4–6 weeks to prevent excessive bending and twisting of the spine. For patients who have developed a foot drop, an ankle foot orthosis (AFO) may be prescribed to allow a better gait pattern.

For patients with brain injury that results in the removal of a portion of the skull, a helmet may be used to protect the brain.

Equipment

Based on the patient's functional improvement, the therapist and physician may prescribe a gait device (rolling walker, hemi walker, platform walker, quad cane, straight cane, etc.) to improve balance during ambulation. In addition, a wheelchair may be prescribed for patients with gait difficulty or poor endurance. Other equipment may include a raised toilet seat, bedside commode, or shower chair to for the patient's safety and independence once home. The occupational therapist may also suggest adaptive equipment (reacher, sock aide, shoe horn, etc.) for those patients with spinal precautions preventing them from bending.

Spasticity

Can occur in patients with either a spinal cord compression/trauma or in those with a brain injury as a result of trauma, tumor, or hemorrhage. Spasticity is defined as an increase in muscle tone which could lead to the development of contractures if aggressive stretching is not done. The role of the therapist is to educate the patient and family on effective stretching techniques. At times, when the spasticity is interfering with function or becomes painful, the physician may start you on oral spasmolytic agents such as baclofen, tizanidine, valium, or dantrium. For those patients where the spasticity is isolated to one specific limb or who cannot tolerate the sedation/dizziness that can occur with oral agents, botulinum toxin injections may be administered into the affected muscle groups. For those who have significant spasticity refractory to oral agents and intramuscular botulinum toxin, the physiatrist or neurologist may discuss placement of an intrathecal baclofen pump system.

Goals/Conclusion

A comprehensive neurorehabilitation program is designed based on identifying problems and setting short and long term goals to address them. The ultimate goal is a holistic approach to restore patients to their previous level of function or as close as possible to the previous level. Not every patient fits neatly into a category. Their team will recommend the post-acute level of care that meets the majority of these patient's needs. It is a lengthy process to achieve the set goals therefore patience is very important while participating actively with the team.

Levels of care	Therapy services	Intensity	Medical
Acute hospital	PT/OT/ST	Evaluation and intensity	High (7 days/week)
Acute hehab	PT/OT/ST	3 h/day, 5–6 days/week	Medium (5–7 days/week
SNF	PT/OT/ST	1–1/2 h/day, 5 days/week	Low (2–3 days/week
LTAC	PT/OT/ST	1 h/day, 3–5 days/week	High (7 days/week)
Outpatient	PT/OT/ST	2–3 times/week/service	Seen in doctor's office
Home health	PT/OT/ST	2–3 times/week/service	Outpatient MD & Home Health Nurse

Pic of PT walking patient (Picture from http://www.houstonmethodist.org/acute-therapies).

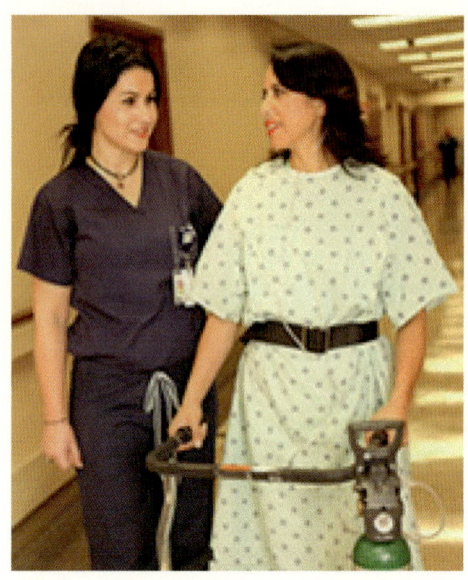

Pic of rehab gym (Picture from http://www.houston-methodist.org/outpatient-rehabilitation).

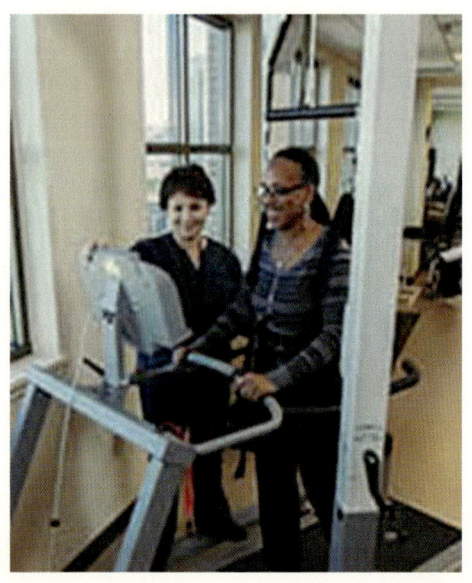

Pic of Equipment (Picture from http://www.stroke-rehab.
com/adaptive-equipment.html).

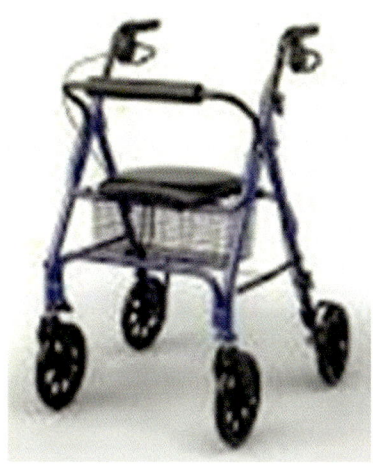

Pic of Bracing AFO (Picture from http://www.medi-
calexpo.com/prod/conwell-medical/ankle-foot-orthoses-
afo-68102-506020.html).

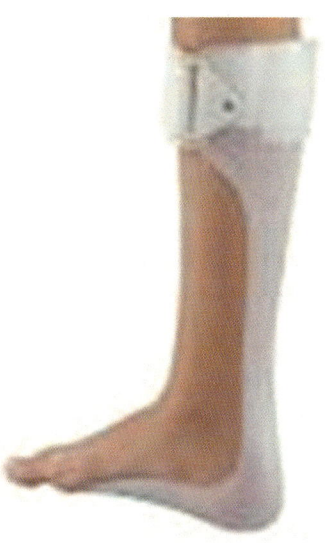

Pic of diagram of CNS and PNS? (Picture from http://www.womens-health-advice.com/nervous-system.html).

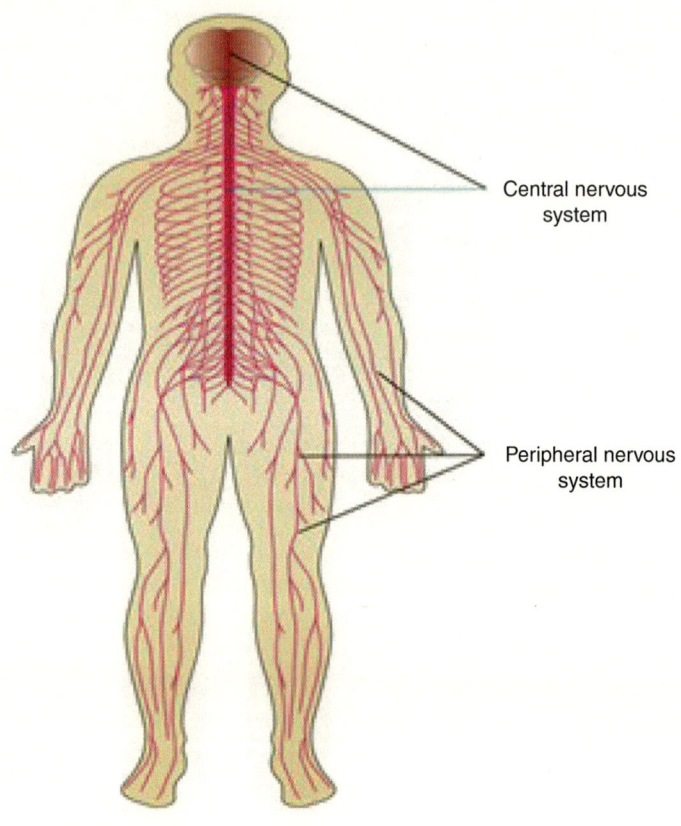

Central nervous system

Peripheral nervous system

Chapter 14
Brain Death

Shahid M. Nimjee

A family member or loved being admitted to the hospital is one of the most difficult times in our lives. There can be fear, anxiety, sadness mixed with uncertainty as to the condition of the patient and their prognosis. No more is this true in the setting of conditions that affect the brain. In the event of a significant brain injury, a patient will not recover despite intervention. While they may look like they are comfortably sleeping while on a ventilator, they may, in fact have lost any meaningful cerebral function. They may be brain dead.

This chapter is meant to provide educate families and friends of patients who are being evaluated for irreversible brain injury. We will cover the medical definition of brain death, how it is clinically evaluated, additional diagnostic studies used to help physicians determine brain and finally, what it means for your loved one.

The definition of brain death is *irreversible arrest of all brain function, including that of the brainstem* [1]. The American Association of Neurology (AAN) first published guidelines in 1995, stating patients who were in a non-responsive state, or coma, had to have a known cause for their

S.M. Nimjee, MD, PhD
Division of Neurosurgery, Department of Radiology,
Duke University Medical Center, Durham, NC 27710, USA
e-mail: shahid.nimjee@duke.edu

A. Agrawal, G. Britz (eds.), *Comprehensive Guide to Neurosurgical Conditions*, DOI 10.1007/978-3-319-06566-3_14, © Springer International Publishing Switzerland 2015

condition, no brainstem and could not breath on their own or have apnea in the absence of a ventilator providing oxygen to their lungs [2]. In 2010, the AAN revised these guidelines to make the complete assessment more conclusive [3]. There are three fundamental sections with items in each that must all be satisfied in order to establish brain death (Table 32.1).

Prerequisites

In order to be evaluated for brain death, the patient must be in a coma of known and irreversible cause. These include ischemic or hemorrhagic stroke, trauma and cerebral herniation. There must be imaging of the brain, either computerized tomography (CT) or magnetic resonance imaging (MRI) scan that can explain the neurological condition.

All drugs that can affect the neurological exam should have been stopped and allowed sufficient time that they have no further impact on the patient. There are some drugs such as neuromuscular blocking agents that can affect evaluation of brain death. The lingering effects these drugs however, can be evaluated with neuromuscular evaluation.

The patient must have a normal body temperature, defined as being greater than or equal to 36 °C. Finally, there should be no derangement in the patient's electrolyte balance, acid–base disturbances in the blood or endocrine dysfunction.

Before beginning the examination, the physician verifies that the patient's blood pressure is greater than 100 mmHg and that they are not spontaneously breathing.

Examination

The physician begins the physical examination by shining a light into the patient's eye to assess pupillary reaction, stimulates the eye, typically with a drop of saline to assess the corneal reflex and move the head with the eyes open to

TABLE 32.1 Brain death checklist

Prerequisites	Examination	Apnea test
Irreversible coma with known cause	No pupillary reaction to light	Hemodynamically stable
Imaging explaining coma	No corneal reflex	Normal carbon dioxide level while on ventilator ($PaCO_2$ 35–45 mmHg)
No CNS depressant drugs	No oculocephalic reflex	Pre-oxygenation with 100 % FiO_2 for greater than 10 min such that PaO_2 is greater than 200 mmHg
No residual muscle relaxing drugs	No oculovestibular reflex	Positive end-expiratory pressure (PEEP) 5 cmH_2O
No severe acid–base, electrolyte or endocrine imbalance	No facial movements to stimulation at eye or temporomandibular joint	Provide oxygen either by suction catheter at the carina at 6 L/min or a connector to endotracheal tube at a continuous positive airway pressure (CPAP) of 10 cmH_2O
Normal body temperature	No gag reflex	
Systolic blood pressure greater than 100 mmHg	No cough when stimulated	
No spontaneous respirations	No limb movement when stimulated	

evaluate the oculocephalic reflex. The examination continues with noxious stimulation of the face to evaluate the facial muscles, which include pressure over the eye (supraorbital pressure), stimulating the nostril (nasopharyngeal pressure) with a suction device or other non-traumatic object or pressure on the jaw joint just in front of the ear (temporo-mandibular pressure). This is then followed by stimulation to the pharynx and trachea.

Pressure exams on the body include pressure on the chest (sternal rub) or pressure on the finger nail beds. This evaluates a cortical response to pain.

Apnea Test

The apnea test evaluates a patient's respiratory drive – the reflex to breath in the setting of too much carbon dioxide (hypercarbia) or acidity in the body. As previously mentioned, the patient must have a systolic blood greater than 100 mmHg to correctly perform this test. The carbon dioxide level must be normal and the patient should be receive enough pressurized oxygen such that the partial pressure is 200 mmHg or more.

The blood carbon dioxide partial pressure is increased to 60 or 20 mmHg greater than normal for that patient. If there is no spontaneous breathing in this setting, the test is concluded to be positive.

There are instances where the evaluation described above still does not have a definitive result or the test itself cannot be adequately performed. In those situations, ancillary tests are performed. These include photon emission tomography nuclear scan (PET), electroencephalogram (EEG), transcranial Doppler ultrasound (TCD) and digital subtraction angiography (DSA).

Photon emission tomography is an imaging study that uses a radionucleotide and uptake by the brain is measured. Lack of uptake occurs in patients who are brain dead.

An electroencephalogram is a measurement of the electrical activity of the brain. In patients who are brain dead, there is no electrical activity above 2 μV and no reaction to audio or visual stimulation.

Transcranial doppler ultrasound is a bedside test where a handheld ultrasound probe can measure the velocity of blood flowing through brain vessels. There is no evidence of blood flow in patients who are brain dead.

Digital subtraction angiography is a procedure where a small sheath is placed in the patient's femoral artery and a catheter is advanced into the carotid and vertebral arteries. Iodine-based contrast is injected under pressure through the catheter in order to view the vessels of the brain. In patients who are brain dead, contrast does not perfuse the brain.

In patients who meet criteria for brain death, a reasonable thought is that they are motionless. Paradoxically, patients who are brain dead can still move as a result of spinal reflexes. In fact, body movement not controlled by the brain occur in between 13 and 75 % of patients who are brain dead [4]. These reflexes include flexing arms and legs, toes pointing downward, facial twitching, myoclonus and a phenomenon known as the *Lazarus sign*. This is where a person who is brain dead will raise both their hands straight up and have them drop across their chest. This complex muscle reflex is confusing and emotionally distressing for family members who witness this, yet does not represent brain activity. Families need to be aware of this possibility and be rest assured that this does not represent spontaneous brain resurgence or an incorrect initial assessment by the medical team.

Determining brain death involves well-trained, experienced physicians, sophisticated equipment and a team of medical support staff in order to efficiently evaluate the patients and report the results. It also involves constant communication with you and your family so that the patient's wishes as you know them are respected and upheld. It is also important that the patient, while at the end of life, continues to be treated with respect and dignity. Finally, this communication is essential to help mitigate your grief, at least somewhat, by understanding this process. We hope that this chapter serves in that capacity.

References

1. Guidelines for the determination of death. Report of the medical consultants on the diagnosis of death to the President's Commission for the Study of Ethical Problems in Medicine and Biomedical and Behavioral Research. JAMA. 1981;246(19):2184–6.
2. Wijdicks EF. Determining brain death in adults. Neurology. 1995;45(5):1003–11.
3. Wijdicks EF, Varelas PN, Gronseth GS, Greer DM. Evidence-based guideline update: determining brain death in adults: report of the Quality Standards Subcommittee of the American Academy of Neurology. Neurology. 2010;74(23):1911–8.
4. Greer DM, Curiale GG. End-of-life and brain death in acute coma and disorders of consciousness. Semin Neurol. 2013;33(2):157–66.

Chapter 15
Organ Donation and the Neurosurgical Patient

John C. Lohlun and Zakiyah Kadry

The only gift is a portion of thyself. ~Ralph Waldo Emerson

The Need for Organs

Each year, more than 7,000 deceased donors make more than 20,000 organ transplants possible [17]. Organs such as the heart, lung, liver, kidneys, pancreas, and small bowel are potentially life-saving. Even tissues such bone, tendons, ligaments, corneas, skin, and heart valves from cadaveric donors can be procured and used to replace such tissues damaged by trauma or disease. However, the need for organs still surpasses availability. As of 2013, more than 110,000 patients of all ages currently await life-saving organ transplants. An average of 18 people die daily because of the lack of organs. Neurosurgical patients who suffer catastrophic intracranial events are a major source of organ donation [5]. This chapter aims to inform families of loved ones who have sustained

J.C. Lohlun (✉) • Z. Kadry
Division of Transplantation, Department of Surgery,
Penn State Hershey Medical Center, Hershey, PA, USA
e-mail: John.Lohlun@baystatehealth.org; zkadry@hmc.psu.edu

A. Agrawal, G. Britz (eds.), *Comprehensive Guide to Neurosurgical Conditions*, DOI 10.1007/978-3-319-06566-3_15, © Springer International Publishing Switzerland 2015

irreversible brain injuries of the process of organ donation, and also to encourage individuals to help alleviate the organ shortage by signing up to be a donor with their state's donor registry.

The OPTN, UNOS, and the OPO

In 1984, the National Organ Transplant Act was passed by the US Congress [4]. The act called for a national Organ Procurement and Transplantation Network (OPTN) to be created. The aim of the OPTN is to manage the country's organ procurement, donation, and transplantation system and to increase the availability of and access to donor organs for patients with end stage organ failure [8, 9]. OPTN members include all US transplant centers, organ procurement organizations (OPO), histocompatibility laboratories, voluntary health care organizations, medical and scientific organizations, and members of the general public. UNOS (United Network for Organ Sharing) currently based in Virginia was awarded the OPTN contract in 1986 by the Health Resources and Services Administration (HRSA) of the U.S. Department of Health and Human Services (HHS). UNOS has operated the OPTN continually since that time under contract with HRSA. The Organ Procurement Organization (OPO) is the local agency responsible for the recovery, preservation and transportation of organs for transplantation. Currently there are 58 OPOs in the US. One of the aims of the OPO is to educate the public about the critical need for organ donation. An OPO's service area can include a portion of a state, an entire state, or more than one state. The OPO will be notified when a patient in a hospital is a potential organ donor. Coordinators from the OPO will then approach the family of the potential donor with the aim of building a rapport with the family during this trying and stressful time and to explain the process of organ donation . When a donor is identified and organs become available for transplantation, an electronic list of potential recipients is generated from the OPO's local service area. If no suitable match is made, a wider regional list of potential recipients is generated, followed by a national list.

Who Can Be a Donor?

Typical neurosurgical patients who are potential organ donors include those who have sustained unrecoverable intracranial cerebrovascular accidents and traumatic brain injuries. Even brain dead patients who have brain tumors may be able to donate organs and tissues provided that their tumors have no malignant potential or have not metastasized. As medical science evolves, donation opportunities change and may widen. A patient's medical condition at the time of death determines which organs and tissues can be donated. Donation does not interfere with medical care. Consent for donation is confirmed by verifying the person's enrollment on a state registry (and typically will be noted on one's drivers license) or by obtaining written consent from the family. The organ procurement procedure is a surgical operation which can take up to 3–4 h, during which the body is treated with the utmost of respect and care. Organ donation will not change or delay funeral arrangements and will not interfere with open casket funeral viewing. It is illegal to buy and sell organs and tissues in the United States, and there is no cost to the deceased donor's family for organ and tissue donation.

Organ Donation by Brain Death

Organ and tissue donation can only occur after all life-saving efforts have been made and death has been declared [2, 7, 15]. During the earliest years of transplantation through the 1960s , determination of death required the heart to stop. The first deceased donor kidney, liver and heart transplants in 1958, 1963, and 1967 respectively were all performed using organs recovered from donors who had irreversible cessation of cardiac and circulatory function (hence the term cardiac death or non-heart beating donors) . In the 1960's, the concept of brain death came into being with the report of the Ad Hoc Committee of the Harvard Medical School in 1968 [1] establishing the criteria for the determination of brain death. Brain death has since been endorsed by all the major medical and legal professional associations in the United States and Europe [13]. Organs procured from brain dead individuals seem to function better than those procured from cardiac death donors , as the latter organs are more exposed to the effects of low blood flow with resulting poor oxygenation of the tissues and consequent poor graft function. For the next quarter of a century, virtually all organ donation was from brain dead individuals. In 2004, only 4 % of deceased donors in the United States were cardiac death donors [16]. Cardiac and pulmonary functions in brain dead individuals are usually intact or maintained with respirators or medications. For this reason, brain death can be emotionally very distressing and puzzling to family and friends, because their loved ones appear warm, alive and viable, but these patients are , in fact, dead. Another source of confusion for family members can be the distinction between brain death and the persistent vegetative state. The latter is defined as a disorder of consciousness in which patients with severe brain damage are in a state of partial arousal rather than true awareness. These patients are not brain dead, and organ procurement from such patients is illegal [7].

Organ Donation by Cardiac Death (Non-heart Beating Donors)

In the last 15 years, there has been renewed interest in the use of organs from cardiac death donors not only to increase the donor pool but also because of increased public and family reluctance to prolong futile treatment and artificial support for their loved ones, and the increased use of advance directives and health care proxies [10, 14, 16, 19,

20]. Transplantation results using organs from cardiac death donors have also improved. In 1993, there were only 42 cardiac death donors, providing 81 organ transplants. In 2003, there were 270 cardiac death donors, providing 549 organs . In 2012, this percentage increased to 14 % (1,106 cardiac death donors providing 1,900 abdominal organ transplants) [18] . These organs are procured usually under controlled conditions after referral of dying patients to the local OPO. These donors are comatose, irreversibly brain-damaged, and ventilator-dependent who are receiving artificial support with virtually no hope of improvement and are not brain-dead by definition. The decision to withdraw supportive care is made by the family and the primary medical team, and appropriate consent is obtained from the family. Respiratory and intravenous pressor support is discontinued in the operating room or intensive care unit, and cardiac function is monitored, and death is pronounced by standard cardiac criteria, either by the absence of a heart beat on auscultation of the heart or the absence of a cardiac rhythm on cardiac monitor. Organ procurement proceeds speedily because, during this time of failing and ultimately absent cardiac and respiratory function, organs are susceptible to the effects of poor or absent oxygenation. The time period between withdrawal of cardiac and respiratory support and certification of cardiac death is termed warm ischemic time. Different organs have different tolerance to warm ischemia, and in some cases these organs can have poor function, primary non-function or significantly increased complication rates after transplantation [14]. For example, the liver tolerates warm ischemic times no longer than 30 min. Kidneys should have a warm ischemic time no longer than 90 min. If cardiac death is not pronounced within these warm ischemia times, these organs will no longer be able to be transplanted. It is also possible that a potential donor remains alive 60–90 min after withdrawal of cardiac and respiratory support. Organ procurement is then aborted and the patient is returned back to the floor for comfort measures only. These patients almost invariably expire in the next few hours. While controlled organ procurement from cardiac death donors is practiced in the USA in the fashion described above, uncontrolled procurement from cardiac death donors is also practiced in some countries, particularly in Europe [3, 12, 21]. These donors sustain circulatory arrest at the scene of an accident, fail to respond to cardiopulmonary resuscitation and are declared dead on arrival at the hospital. Because organ procurement is somewhat unplanned, these organs suffer severe protracted ischemia before recovery, and transplantation of such organs have produced mixed results.

References

1. A definition of irreversible coma: report of the Ad hoc Committee of the Harvard Medical School to examine the definition of brain death. JAMA. 1968;205:337–40.
2. Beaucham T, Childress J. Principle of biomedical ethics. 7th ed. New York: Oxford University Press; 2012.
3. Bonnie RJ, Wright S, Dineen KK. Legal authority to preserve organs in cases of uncontrolled cardiac death: preserving family choice. J Law Med Ethics. 2008;36(4):741–51.
4. Department of Health and Human Services. Organ Procurement and Transplantation Network: Final Rule. 42 CFR, Section 121. Available from: http://optn.transplant.hrsa.gov/policiesAndBylaws/final_rule.asp.
5. Dickerson J, Valadka AB, et al. Organ donation rates in a neurosurgical intensive care unit. J Neurosurg. 2002;97(4):811–4.
6. Freeman RB, Cohen JT. Transplantation risks and the real world: what does 'high risk' really mean? Am J Transplant. 2009; 9(1):23–30.
7. Jonsen AR. The god squad and the origins of transplantation ethics and policy. J Law Med Ethics. 2007;35(2):238–40.
8. Klein AS, Messersmith EE, Ratner LE, Kochik R, Baliga PK, Ojo AO. Organ donation and utilization in the United States, 1999-2008. Am J Transplant. 2010;10(4 Pt 2):973–86.
9. McDiarmid SV, Pruett TL, Graham WK. The oversight of solid organ transplantation in the United States. Am J Transplant. 2008;8:739–44.
10. Merion RM, Pelletier SJ, Goodrich N, Englesbe MJ, Delmonico FL. Donation after cardiac death as a strategy to increase deceased donor liver availability. Ann Surg. 2006;244(4):555–62.

11. National Organ Transplant Act, 42 United States Code, Section 273, available from: http://optn.transplant.hrsa.gov/policiesAndBylaws/nota.asp.
12. Otero A, Gomez-Gutierrez M, Suarez F, et al. Liver transplantation from Maastricht category 2 non-heartbeating donors. Transplantation. 2003;76:1068–73.
13. Quality standards sub-committee of the American Academy of Neurology. Practice parameters for determining brain death in adults (summary statement). Neurology. 1995;45(5):1012–14.
14. Reich DJ, Mulligan DC, Abt PL, Pruett TL, Abecassis MM, D'Alessandro A, et al. ASTS recommended practice guidelines for controlled donation after cardiac death organ procurement and transplantation. Am J Transplant. 2009;9(9):2004–11.
15. Report of the medical consultants on the diagnosis of death to the president's commission for the study of ethical problems in medicine and biomedical and behavioral research. Guidelines for the determination of death. JAMA. 1981;246(19):2184–6.
16. United Network of Organ Sharing. Donation after cardiac death. A reference guide. Richmond; 2004.
17. Talking about transplantation. UNOS website (available online at http://www.unos.org/index.php). 2013.
18. Unpublished data. UNOS. Richmond; 2013
19. US Institute of Medicine. Non-heart-beating organ transplantation: medical and ethical issues in procurement. National Academy Press. Available on-line at www.nap.edu; 1997.
20. US Institute of Medicine. Non-heart-beating organ transplantation: practice and protocols. National Academy Press. Available on-line at www.nap.edu; 2000.
21. Verheijde JL, Rady MY, McGregor J. Presumed consent for organ preservation in uncontrolled donation after cardiac death in the United States: a public policy with serious consequences. Philos Ethics Humanit Med. 2009;4:15.

Chapter 16
Second Opinions from the Perspective of the Patient and the Physician

Robert G. Grossman

Contemplating surgery on one's brain or spine is particularly stressful and likely to be more so than the prospect of abdominal surgery with which most individuals are familiar.

Questions that immediately arise are:

1. Is the surgery necessary-Are there medical alternatives? What will happen if I don't have the operation?
2. What are the complications that can occur and how often do they occur?
3. What are the numbers of successful outcomes?
4. What is the experience and the track record of the surgeon?
5. Is the facility at which the surgery will be done equipped for the procedure?
6. How long will I be in the hospital? When can I return to normal activities and return to work?
7. What is the cost – Radiology, anesthesiology, pathology, hospital charges, surgeon's fee?

In addition to these basic questions there are additional points to consider. There is a natural tendency to fixate on the surgeon but it is also important to consider the team and the

R.G. Grossman, MD
Department of Neurosurgery, Houston Methodist Hospital,
6560 Fannin, Suite 944, Houston, TX 77030, USA
e-mail: rgrossman@houstonmethodist.org

A. Agrawal, G. Britz (eds.), *Comprehensive Guide to Neurosurgical Conditions*, DOI 10.1007/978-3-319-06566-3_16,
© Springer International Publishing Switzerland 2015

facilities that support the surgeon, particularly for major procedures such as intracranial tumors and aneurysms and complex spine surgery with instrumentation. The team and the facilities play an important role in the successful performance of complex Neurosurgery. Consideration should be given to:

1. The availability of anesthesiologists with experience in neuroanesthesia
2. Dedicated neuroradiologists
3. Availability of monitoring the electrical activity of motor and sensory pathways in the spinal cord and brain when appropriate for the surgery
4. Use of image – guided surgery when appropriate
5. For brain and spinal cord tumors, the availability of a neuropathologist to read intraoperative frozen sections of the pathology to determine if the tumor is malignant
6. A dedicated Neurosurgical intensive care unit for postoperative care with dedicated Neuro – intensivists
7. Availability of 24 h in -hospital coverage by Neurosurgical residents

As a patient contemplating surgery you should feel free to ask your surgeon these questions.

You should also consider your surgeon's approach to you as an individual.

Did your surgeon:

1. Take a detailed history of your symptoms and the course of the development of your illness?
2. Perform a detailed physical and neurological examination?
3. Review your x-rays and scans with you showing you the pathology and explaining how it was causing your symptoms?
4. Explain the recommended surgery and mention alternative surgical approaches and the reasons for choosing the recommended approach?
5. Give you contact numbers and offer to talk to relevant family members and others who may not have been present at the time of your visit?

6. Will your surgeon have a long-term medical relationship with you including follow-up examinations and reviewing your x-rays and scans over the years following surgery If your condition is such that it requires follow-up as in the case of brain tumors?

If you, as the patient, feel that the surgeon has the capability and the concern for you to provide the best treatment, a second opinion is likely to be superfluous. Uncertainty is an indication to obtain a second opinion. Patients are often reluctant to tell a surgeon that they would like a second opinion. Anxiety should not inhibit you from requesting a second opinion. A sensible surgeon will welcome a second opinion, particularly in cases where there is considerable risk of impairment following surgery. Patients may also be reluctant to tell the surgeon giving a second opinion that it is only a second opinion and that they will have the procedure done by the initial surgeon that they have seen. Pre-approvals required by insurance companies for physician's visits that specify the service to be performed at the visit make this scenario less likely to occur today than in the past. Openness is the best policy. You, as the patient, should look for the same thoroughness in history taking, review of the records and neurological examination as would be expected from the initial physician.

The physician giving a second opinion should recognize that an opinion that differs from that of the initial opinion is often upsetting and confusing to the patient. Before delivering your opinion it is helpful to ask the patient "What is your understanding of what Dr.____ has told you about your condition and what procedures and treatment have been recommended?" The patient's answers to this question will provide the data that you need to give an appropriate explanation and recommendation if you differ from the primary opinion or enable you to definitively assent to the primary opinion.

It is hoped that these thoughts will provide guidance to patients and physicians considering what to look for in and how to conduct a second opinion.

Chapter 17
Nursing Perspectives

Kathryn Kerrigan

Before Your Visit

You have been referred to a specialist and have made an appointment. Before your scheduled visit make arrangements for you records, including radiology reports, to be sent to your neurosurgeon and plan to have copies of CT and MRI images available for review. Plan to attend your visit with a family member or friend, this support person can help you take notes and remember instructions. Your specialist may have health history forms that will need to be filled out for your visit. When possible, have the office e-mail or send you the forms so they can be filled out ahead of time. An accurate history of the duration of you symptoms, the aggravating and alleviating factors, and previous treatments will help your surgeon determine your plan. If surgery is to be scheduled, your surgeon will need to know all of the medications you are taking, including over the counter and herbal medications, as some of these may need to be stopped prior to a surgery or procedure to prevent increased bleeding and interactions with anesthesia.

K. Kerrigan, MSN, FNP-BC
Houston Methodist Neurological Institute,
6560 Fannin, Suite 944, Houston, Texas 77030, USA
e-mail: kmkerrigan@houstonmethodist.org

A. Agrawal, G. Britz (eds.), *Comprehensive Guide to Neurosurgical Conditions*, DOI 10.1007/978-3-319-06566-3_17, © Springer International Publishing Switzerland 2015

In addition to the office visit with your surgeon, patients may need preoperative consults with cardiology or anesthesia prior to admission. During the time between your clinic visit and scheduled surgery, keep your surgeon updated on any changes in your symptoms. Patients with fever, productive cough or active infection may need to have elective procedures rescheduled in order to allow time for treatment.

For the Hospitalized Patient

Patients are admitted to a unit based on stability and the complexity of monitoring they need and may transition through multiple inpatient and observation units before discharge. Your nurse will help orient you to your hospital room and explain any unit specific policies for visitors.

While there is no typical day for a neurosurgical patient, you can expect to have the following as part of your routine. A nurse or other member of the healthcare team will assess your vital signs; temperature, respiratory rate, pulse, blood pressure and pain level. In addition to a general physical examination, a neurological assessment is performed to assess level of consciousness, pupillary signs, and motor tone and strength. The extent and frequency of the exam will vary with condition and the stability of the patient.

During an inpatient stay your diet and medications will be prescribed and provided by the hospital. Diets are based on the ability to swallow and tolerate solid foods and meals may be timed around tests and procedures to prevent aspiration. Please check with your nurse before bringing outside food to a patient.

You can expect to see your neurosurgeon or hospitalist at least one each day. These visits are not easily timed as surgeons may round between cases. It's easy to forget your questions when the doctor stops by unexpectedly, write down any questions you may have so that they may be addressed during rounds.

Preparing for Discharge

Your discharge location will depend on your needs and preferences.

Make sure you understand the reason for your hospitalization and what signs and symptoms to look out for during your recovery at home. In addition to changes in neurological status, you should be monitoring for worsening pain, fever, and shortness of breath. Patients should know what to look out for and how to reach their surgeon if questions or concerns arise after discharge.

If you were hospitalized for surgery, you may have an incision to care for. Follow only your surgeon's instructions on when you can shower and what, if any, medications need to be applied to the healing area. Generally, if the wound was closed with staples or sutures, these are removed after 7–10 days.

You should be provided with clear instructions for taking any medications, especially new medications, at the time of discharge. If you were instructed to stop taking blood thinners prior to a scheduled surgery, you will be given instructions or should ask when these can be safely resumed. Some patients will be prescribed blood thinners as part of the medical management for stroke, intracranial stenosis, or after endovascular flow diversion for aneurysm treatment. Herbal and some over the counter medications have the potential to interact with blood thinners and other prescribed medications. Check with your doctor or hospital pharmacist before resuming or adding herbal and over the counter medications to you regimen.

Patients may have been seen by a number of specialists during a hospitalization and follow-up clinic appointments and tests may need to be scheduled after discharge. Make arrangements for your hospital records and test results to be sent to your primary care provider for continuity of care.

For the Family

You are the advocate during the hospital stay and the care provider for patients who may not be ready to completely care for themselves after discharge. Never be afraid to speak up if you do not understand a diagnosis or treatment plan. Get involved early in helping your loved one with meals, physical therapy, and personal care if needed. You play an important role in ensuring that your loved one receives the care they need and it is equally important for you to do the same for yourself.

Index

A. Agrawal, G. Britz (eds.), *Comprehensive Guide to
Neurosurgical Conditions*, DOI 10.1007/978-3-319-06566-3,
© Springer International Publishing Switzerland 2015

Printed by Printforce, the Netherlands